Take Charge
of Your **Health**

A Biblical Perspective

Lilli Taylor Hetherington

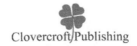

Clovercroft Publishing

Take Charge of Your Health: A Biblical Perspective

©2014 by Lilli Taylor Hetherington

Published by Clovercroft Publishing, Franklin, Tennessee

Published in association with Larry Carpenter of Christian Book Services, LLC
www.christianbookservices.com

Interior Layout Design by Suzanne Lawing

Edited by Andrew Toy

Printed in the United States of America

978-1-940262-63-5

What Christian Leaders Have to Say about Lilli Hetherington and *Take Charge of Your Health – A Biblical Perspective*

"Lilli Hetherington has been a very inspirational guest on our show, *Life Today*. The material she presents is greatly needed and in high demand, but *few* offer such sound, sensible advice. Lilli has thoroughly researched the Scriptures and has a keen awareness of how to apply these principles in a biblical way. The negative effect poor nutrition is having on our bodies is a major cause of the illnesses we experience today. Lilli gives real hope in turning this process around."
- JAMES ROBISON, *Life Today TV*, Life Outreach International

"I am glad Lilli is offering her knowledge about such a needed area of our lives . . . she is helping us to face honestly the stewardship of our bodies."
- DUDLEY HALL, Kerygma Ventures

"God, the creator of our bodies, knows the power secrets for making them function efficiently. Lilli Hetherington reminds us of God's guidelines in the Scriptures, laying out a simple plan for healthy living. Isn't it fascinating that scientific research is now becoming aware of these very same principles that God told us from the beginning? The ministry Lilli offers challenges me to take a closer look at God's Word and the food choices set before me. I've made rewarding and satisfying changes in the process of applying what I've learned."
- JEANNE ROGERS, *Life Today TV* with James Robison, Life Outreach International

"The body of Christ certainly needs the message Lilli is offering."
- CHERYL TOWNSLEY, Lifestyle for Health

"As Christians, our goal should be to be like Christ. Many people just focus on the spiritual aspects of that goal, yet there are physical responsibilities as well. Doing your best nutritionally to take care of your body is just as important as nurturing your spirit for God's purpose for our lives on this earth. I believe Lilli Hetherington is powerfully called to help people fulfill this aspect of the Christian life—divine health. I encourage you to listen to what she has to say. I believe God has entrusted Lilli with a message that is absolutely relevant for today."
- PASTOR AMY HOSSLER, Covenant Church, Carrollton, Texas

"Lilli has been affiliated with our radio station since we signed on many years ago. She is a huge asset as a spokeswoman for health through this arena. Personally, she has been my incredible 'health coach' for many years. Lilli is extremely knowledgeable in helping me know what foods to avoid in my diet and what things to add as I get older. Applying knowledge from this book to our lives can help guarantee our being strong and healthy for the long haul!"
- KAY JONES, 100.7 FM, KWRD, Salem Communications

Contents

Preface

In our United States we have the best of medical care in the whole world . . . we desperately need it!

In the Christian community, we have the best prayer warriors in the whole world . . . we desperately need them!

With that gratefully said, why do we still lead the world in sickness and disease ranking 150th in world health?

For example, breast cancer is a huge issue for women in the United States. More than two hundred thousand cases are diagnosed every year. Should we only be treating cancer once it's diagnosed? Thank God for "early detection," but is there anything women can do to protect themselves from ever getting this awful disease prior to diagnosis? What are some natural preventative steps that women can take to help keep themselves healthy?

Thankfully, this book answers those very important questions.

In our family, any time we have encountered a health crisis, we have engaged the best medical advice, faithful prayer warriors, and good nutrition. This approach has always been a win-win!

Who Can Benefit from this Book? From the Cradle to the Grave

Cradle: Why does a child born in Shanghai have a better chance of living a long and healthy life than a child born in the US?

Children: The number one killer of children, next to accidents, is cancer.

Seniors: The elderly are dying in their seventies on a long list of pharmaceuticals from long and lingering illnesses.

Everything You Need to Know about Healthy Nutrition and Have Not Been Taught!

What sets this book apart from the other thousands of books on nutrition? *With the plethora of books on nutrition, why are we still experiencing a million heart attacks a year, one-half million to cancer, and why is diabetes taking our nation to the brink?* This is a tsunami of sickness and disease. *To further illustrate, we spend two trillion dollars a year fighting and managing our sickness.* Two trillion on disease is four times the entire defense budget. *We spend more on disease* than we do on food, defense, and housing combined every year. This book answers all of these "why" questions. Most of the information we read is simply not getting to the root cause.

Where Is the Outcry?

This is the message *that is missing* in all of our equipping. How many messages have you heard on this topic? It's sad the average Christian can sit in the average church his entire lifetime and not hear one message from the pulpit on how take charge of his temple. Yet 90 percent of church prayer requests are for healing of preventable diseases in our physical body.

This is profoundly sad.

Many do not know that *God has a grocery list . . . and it is perfect. It was and still is.* His groceries have everything we need to prevent this entire epidemic of disease. The good news is when we eat God's grocery list, the following can happen:

> *"He blesses my mouth with good things."*
> *Eating this way can add twenty-nine years of good life.*
> *My body is able to reproduce a new liver in just six months (can't live without a liver!).*
> *My body cells are able to reproduce and become totally new in just eleven months.*
> *Every ounce of bone in the body can become totally new in just two years (which means you don't need to die from a hip fracture).*

It's curious that as a nation, we lead the world in osteoporosis and osteopenia and we drink more cow's milk than any other nation. Isn't that interesting! The Dairy Council is not readily volunteering that statistic.

This book tells you simply what to eat to avoid cancer, heart disease, and all of the other top killers and what not to eat if you do not want cancer. Most Americans do not have this knowledge. From reading this book, you will know exactly what causes and cures cancer. **It is no mystery.** So if you are breathless from running for a cure, you can take in a deep breath and stop running (unless you just want to run for your own good health). We know the cure for cancer and all of the other degenerative diseases. It was given to us four thousand years ago, but sadly, it is not being taught. This book is not just called *Take Charge of Your Health,* but rather *Take Charge of Your Health – a Biblical Perspective.* With the status of health as it is today, we need a fresh paradigm or perspective on this subject.

With the thousands of nutrition books on the shelves of bookstores today, why are we still experiencing one million heart attacks *every year* in our nation? Why are twenty thousand people dying of cancer *every day* and one-half million still dying of cancer every year? Why do more than 370 million people have diabetes? *These diseases are all about nutrition.* This book answers those questions and is the missing part in all of our equipping. Yet, it is a top priority to God. One of His first commands was for His children to eat a certain grocery list to live long, healthy lives on earth. His grocery list is anti-inflammatory. Inflammation is a huge cause of these diseases that are killing Americans. Isn't it interesting that the world's grocery list is pro-inflammatory? Have you ever noticed the pro-inflammatory foods in the grocery carts of people standing in line at the pharmaceutical counter waiting to fill their prescriptions and get their toxic-filled flu shots? We can connect some dots here that maybe the very foods they are eating are producing inflammation in their bodies. It's no wonder they are sick and needing pharmaceuticals . . . which then make them even sicker.

When people have heart attacks, they often begin to think about their diet and how it needs to change in order to avoid another heart attack. *It is noteworthy that it has taken seven years of eating a poor diet before heart disease and cancer can even be diagnosed.* How much better it would have been to have been on a program of prevention. Assuming that their disease just flew in the window and they caught it, many have not made the connection that what they are eating three meals a day is causing their sickness. You can read more about the status of the health of our nation in the chapter entitled "What Is the Status of Health in America Today?" What is missing in our equipping? Something surely is missing that matters.

One of the Bible's most beautiful truths is about the food that is good for us (these are the colorful foods like the colors in the rainbow) in addition to the foods we should avoid if we want to walk in health and experience a long and satisfying life and *not die prematurely.* The Bible is quite a manual for nutrition. Isn't it profoundly sad we are not being taught nutrition from God's nutrition manual? When our cars don't work, we check the manual or take them to an expert who fixes them *according to the manual.*

According to the Bible, God promises every human being 120 years of life when we are eating right and our lifestyle lines up with His best. In Exodus 15:26 He says, "If you will diligently listen and obey Me, I will be your health." When those conditions are met, a human lifespan of 120 years is pretty well guaranteed. Most of us have been led to believe what is written in Psalm 90:10, "The days of our years are three-score and ten" (70 years). However, this was written to a rebellious people. The footnote in most translations states, "This was considered to be a curse; God intended man to live 120 years." God's heart is for His people to live and be blessed with a fruitful 120 years of life. This verse in Genesis 6:3 exceeds Psalms 90:10. And *WOW*: He has even told us how.

It is profoundly sad that the average Christian can sit in the average church his entire lifetime and not hear one message from the pulpit on how to take charge of his temple (the human body). Yet, 90 percent of the needs and prayer requests in the church are for healing of disease in our human body. We are being taught many wonderful topics in the church. We learn how to pray effectively, how to witness, how to be a strong missionary, how to be a spirit-filled Christian, how to experience the love of the Father, and how to handle finances. But as important as these subjects truly are, what if you drop dead suddenly and prematurely of a heart attack in your fifties, sixties, or seventies? What if you are diagnosed with preventable cancer because you had not been taught, and you die a premature death? These diseases dramatically disrupt your life forever. *Your ministry is shortened.* Now, you don't feel like praying so much or witnessing, and even walking in the spirit can be a challenge. At this point, you may struggle with the love of the Father thinking He could have prevented your disease. We often blame God when we get sick. You feel bad, you ache all over, and that's all you can think about. How beneficial are all of these other subjects you have been studying if you did not know that the foods you are eating three times a day are the very ones that have made you sick and may take you out prematurely? God has instructed us to not eat certain types of animals, for example, and if you eat them, He guarantees an abomination of disease and premature death.

Americans eat a million animals an hour. Wow! That's a whole lot of dead animals! You can read more about this in the chapter entitled "Foods that Kill." For example, sadly, many Christians are eating the most unholy meat there is on the most holy day of the year, Easter. Most have not heard the truth about how the animal they ate for Easter is full of disease and parasites (this is the day we are celebrating life and resurrection). Many have believed the lie that because we are under grace, we can eat whatever we want. If prayer and grace alone were all we needed for our health, we would be one of the healthiest nations in the world, but we are one of the sickest. Why? There's more we need than healing prayer and the message of grace. **<u>A very powerful spiritual weapon</u>** God has given us against disease is a *healthy grocery list*. That is what this book is all about.

The diseases that are killing us in our nation are not due to our genetics. Nor are these diseases flying in the window or sitting next to us on a plane where we could "catch" them. They are ones for which we cannot be immunized. They are coming from what we are putting in our bodies three meals a day. But it is for lack of knowledge God's people are perishing (Hosea 4:6). We are not being taught God's original health plan.

This is very sad to me. God's health plan costs much less than the world's health plan or schemes. And it is a thousand times more enjoyable. Honestly, how fun is it really to have to hang out at hospitals and doctor's offices because you are sick? Do you really love all those pharmaceuticals that mask your sickness and cause other diseases? Do you just love those ungodly side effects? Do you really love swelling of the lips, tongue, and foaming at the mouth . . . not to mention death as a potential side effect. I believe believers deserve to be informed on this topic.

God's heart of compassion is so well expressed in 3 John 1:2, which states, "I wish above everything else that you would prosper and be in health as your soul prospers." It was and still is a priority to God because He knows that a well-functioning mind and body are essential to fulfilling our assignments. This book is a tool that can prosper your mind, will, and emotions on what foods to eat and what foods to avoid to live a long, satisfying, and preferable life. It is time for believers to *KNOW* the truth about what is killing us. I encourage you to read more about the long and productive lives of other cultures in the chapter entitled "Other Cultures."

Something is missing and what is missing really does matter a whole lot and is in this book. I hope that it will bless you and extend your life to be years worth living. And with the status of health in our nation, this information is so very timely.

I have been sick and I have been well, and I like "well" better! So let's learn how to "be well" (3 John 1:2). I wish above all else that you "be well" as your soul prospers (Improvised edition). Our thirsty souls need to be taught how to be well as never before.

Deep Appreciation

With deep appreciation to my *wonderful* husband, James Hetherington, my greatest encourager and "critic" who has given me his constant encouragement, support, devoted assistance, and most of all, his unconditional love for many years. Your unconditional love has been used for deep healing of my value as a woman. I love you and deeply appreciate you more than you could begin to imagine.

I want to acknowledge my two sons, Brent and Barry, who had the benefits of this nutritional plan from the womb. They honestly came out of the womb doing "push-ups!" They did a heroic job of cooperating with these nutritional guidelines as they were growing up. The years where you were still "in the nest" were the best years of my life. I love you and appreciate who you have turned out to be more than you could ever imagine.

I also want to acknowledge deep appreciation for a wonderful colleague in this field, Dr. Bruce Miller. Dr. Miller is a certified nutrition specialist and a member of the American College of Nutrition. He is the author of many nutritional booklets and *The Nutrition Guarantee.* Dr. Miller's impressive credentials are a mile long. Mainly, I deeply appreciate the constant support he has provided me in this field. His guidance when I was poisoned on a health product was instrumental in saving my life—and therefore, has benefited thousands.

Did You Know?

THE BODY OF CHRIST IS IN A HUGE HEALTH CRISIS!

Have you noticed?

If so, it must sadden you as it does me.

It's a crisis we dare not ignore any longer!

Far too many have believed the myth that sickness is inevitable.

The information in this book is extraordinary, and we don't hear it often enough.

Yet it is easy to understand and to put into practice.

Observations . . . not judgments:

> The body of Christ is not feeling well.
> The body of Christ is tired.
> The body of Christ is physically sick.

Oh, but it doesn't need to be this way.

For many, it is difficult to stand during the entire worship service due to prematurely weak knees, hips, and joints. This is caused by inflammation and crystallization in the joints, muscles, and tendons. You might say, "Isn't that just a normal part of aging?" This picture is far too common, but it is *not* normal, and it is not from aging. Or can we blame these symptoms on having been given "bad genes?" Science tells us that 20 percent of our health is due to the genetic card we have been dealt, but 80 percent is due to our lifestyle choices. You may not be able to do anything about your genetics, but you **can** change your bio terrain internally, and you **can** change your thinking and eating habits **if** you have the correct information. Simply stated, these symptoms are avoidable, preventable, and within our control. When the body gets what it needs, it will do you well. Your body is always trying to maintain a state of wellness. Your body was made to heal itself. Now, as I see it, that is GOOD NEWS. Disease doesn't just "fly in the window." I do believe most want to eat right and think right but due to wrong training, upbringing, and incorrect information, they simply don't know how. I have good news for you and can promise you that this book will tell you how.

Do You Know How?

Here is an interesting piece of information. I have been affiliated with an incredibly outstanding Christian radio station for years. So the people who typically seek my counsel are wonderfully Word-filled, faith-filled, and Spirit-filled believers. But not one person who has sought my counsel for their health issues had been eating the Bible-prevention eating plan. Most have not even known there *is* a biblical nutritional plan that prevents, for example, cancer. All of these well-educated believers and even scholars have not had a clue that what they eat or don't eat is very, very important to God and has *everything to do with whether they live or die.* They have been looking to the Bible for everything else, *but not for their groceries.* Many would think the subject of groceries not very spiritual at all, yet it is a top priority to God. He says in 3 John 1:2: "I wish above everything else that you would prosper and be in health as your soul prospers.

Some say, "Well, praise the Lord for early detection." However, prevention is of far superior value to early detection. But I believe we can be thankful for both.

It Is Sad God's People Have Not Been Taught That If They Neglect the Physical Part, It Will Break Down No Matter How Spiritual We Are

It is a law. We can't trick the God-made system by saying, "I am just running on the Spirit, prayer, or even the Word." *That sounds so spiritual,* but our bodies have not yet been redeemed. They still run on physical laws. Jesus told us in Matthew 5 that the physical laws are with us until the end of the age. And this is true whether we are faith-filled, Word-filled, and Spirit-filled believers.

Are You Worried about Suffering from a Long and Lingering Illness?

Here is what is happening far too often. Many are subconsciously or consciously embracing the "three score and ten" lifespan and giving up at age seventy. It's subtle. If for most of our lives we have not been giving the body what it needs, we begin to get sick with degenerative diseases at three-score and ten. Many think this is just normal. Research indicates that by the time most people reach seventy in our nation, they are on at least five medications a day. And, oh my goodness—there's a better way! The cells of the body begin to degenerate. Sadly, I have a lot of friends and family in this category. I can only help those who seek my help with an open mind. Degenerative diseases are coming from what we put into our bodies. They are diseases like heart conditions, strokes, cancer, diabetes, osteoporosis, arthritis, and many others. But is this God's plan? Three score and ten is considered to be a curse (it was written to a people who were disobedient); God intended man to live to 120 without disease. **We don't have to get sick in order to die.** We will be covering a lot more about this later in the book, and we'll discuss how great it is that we don't have to *suffer* from long and lingering illnesses in order to leave this world.

The reality is that we are losing one million people a year to preventable heart disease and one-half million people to preventable cancer. Preventable means that God has given us the keys and guidelines to not ever have heart disease, strokes, cancer, diabetes, or any other degenerative disease. These should be foreign to us. If you have embraced the world's system of health, being sick may seem normal to you. But we are doing this to ourselves. These diseases are coming from what we put into our bodies. We can make better and wiser choices. There is something we are believing, saying, eating, doing, or even just thinking that is not in our best interests. I always believe the body is trying to get our attention by saying, "I need your cooperative help to stay well for you."

Isn't It Sad That Believers Are Dying "Foolish" Deaths! Why Do I Say "Foolish" Deaths?

King David said of Abner, "Abner died a foolish death because he stepped out of his boundary of protection" (2 Samuel 3:33). We are doing the same in the name of grace when it comes to our health and what we eat or don't eat. God has given us guidelines and boundaries for a healthy lifestyle. I ask the question, can we eat whatever we want as long as we pray over it? Can we eat whatever we want since we are no longer under a law for salvation? So often, we are praying over and asking God to bless food He said would be a curse if eaten.

We should pray over and about everything without ceasing, but *prayer alone is not enough, and that is the essence of this book.*

When we get sick, the Christian community begins to pray for healing. Praise God for prayer, but there simply are some things we can't *just pray* away. We should always pray, teach, admonish, and prophesy. And we should also give the human body (the temple of the Holy Spirit) what it was designed to have for walking in optimal health for a long and satisfied life. If we are not doing that, we are sick and prematurely dying. *I have been in gatherings where people were praying for the sick and then taking a lunch break to eat the very foods God told us will make us sick!* We do this mindlessly. Why? I believe it is because we have no idea how the foods we are eating impact our health. Many who are very spiritually minded have neglected the physical temple and are out of balance in their physical body. Far too many are in denial as to the impact that mindset is having on their health.

The Church Is In for a Season of Change

Lately, I have been hearing many sound, prophetic voices declare that there is a hundredfold movement coming in the body of Christ soon, and the Church is having to get ready for this harvest. And we must get ready in spirit, soul, and BODY. We certainly need God's enablement to do so. The Kingdom of God is advancing; the season of readiness is passing, and we have some catching up to do. It's almost like we have to get ready on the run. So many who are fortified spiritually are not in shape physically to be able to carry the load that is and will be needed. But you can. The information on how to do that is in these pages for you.

The original mandate in Genesis 1:26, 27 is to take dominion on the earth. We hear a lot of sermons on that, but how are we going to accomplish it without knowing **the original health plan mandate?** The original health plan mandate follows closely in Genesis 1:29, 30. It is a grocery list God commands us to eat in order to have the strength we need in order to take dominion. How many believers are eating from this list? He did not just give us "permission," but rather a *command* on what to eat for long life, health, strength, and vitality. We hear almost nothing about this, yet we need to be eating God's diet plan as if our life depended on it. Why? Because it *does*! Genesis 1:29, 30 (fresh fruits, fresh vegetables, whole grains, raw nuts, and raw seeds) should be our staple. That does not mean you have to be a vegetarian unless you want to be, but this should be your staple (see later chapters for specifics). Many are mindlessly putting junk and pure garbage into their temples that creates a climate of disease. Therefore, we are very sick and weak. But we don't have to be. Later in the book, there are lists of what these foods are . . . which ones we should eat and which ones we should avoid forever unless we want to be sick.

From Genesis to Revelation there are *six hundred* scriptures pertaining to the physical health of the body and living a long, satisfied life. I have listed several toward the end of this book in the chapter entitled "The Benefits of Choosing Life." How many sermons have you heard on this subject? I have heard pastors say that their congregation does not want to hear this message, so they don't teach it. But is that good leadership and shepherding? By default, your people are sick and dying prematurely. As one who has been in the body of Christ in nearly every denomination for over sixty years, I can tell you that most believers have no idea what to eat to not get sick. Far too many pastors and the sheep under their care are dying prematurely of prostate cancer, strokes, and heart attacks purely because they do not know. A pastor cannot teach what he himself is not experiencing. Most are not trained in this subject. But, as never before, this is the time to take charge of our own health.

WE DO NOT NEED TO LOSE ONE MORE GENERAL OR BE-LIEVER IN THE BODY OF CHRIST TO CANCER, HEART DIS-EASE, STROKES, AND DIABETES. EVERYONE OF US IS NEED-ED FOR KINGDOM PURPOSES!

Where Is the End Time Army for the End Time Battles Ahead?

The final generation of the church age will be the most militant Christians to have ever lived. This army of the Lord is described by the prophet Joel as "A people come great and strong, the likes of whom has never been" (Joel 2:2).

Are you prepared to meet the demands that these perilous times hold? Or are you preparing to slow down or even stop at three score and ten, which was considered to be a curse? You don't have to slow down or stop. Are you ready to be the army that God wants all of us to be for the exploits prepared before the foundation of the world? Are you ready to help others and stand in the gap for them?

You will need to be strong in body, soul, and spirit. First Thessalonians 5:23 says, "NOW may the God of peace Himself sanctify you entirely and may your spirit, soul and *body* be preserved complete and whole (with peace in each part), without blame, at the coming of the Lord Jesus Christ." God gave us bodies to be His instruments. How is your body holding up? It is not selfish to take care of, love, and nourish the body God gave you. You are the only one who can do it for you. After all, it is God's house and temple, and He put you in charge.

If you have bought into the world's system that sickness and obesity is somewhat normal and you are living on medications and eating the standard American diet, *you will not* live out your number of days. You are believing and living out a lie, because medications only address the symptoms, not the cause. The cause of your sickness is not being addressed. The world's medicines do not produce health and longevity.

God Took Him Home Early

Do you ever hear this from God's people? "I guess God needed his company and just decided to take him home early." I heard this from a pastor, and it was said about a forty-year-old young man who died of preventable cancer and had a beautiful wife and several children. How do you think that family is going to perceive God? God doesn't take you home prematurely due to cancer because He decides He needs your company. That kind of thinking is foolish thinking. But I have heard this often from believers and pastors. "I guess it was just God's will to call him home" No . . . we are taking *ourselves* out. And many times due to lack of proper knowledge. Let's not blame our premature, diseased deaths on a loving God who wishes above everything else that we prosper and be in health and live long and satisfying lives.

I know people who, because they have not been living the Bible prevention diet, are sick. That is exactly what happens. I have heard many of these same people say, "I guess it's just God's sovereign will and plan to take me home," or "I guess it is just God's will for me to be sick and suffer." That mindset sounds very spiritual but does not line up with God's will and Word. Sometimes we are making statements like these when we don't have any solid answers and don't know what else to say. Let's not blame our sickness on a loving God. We need to blame sickness and premature death on what it really is. It is something for which each of us must take responsibility. The Scripture says, "A curse without a cause does not alight" (Proverbs 26:2) and "Know ye not that your body is the temple of the Holy Spirit; therefore, take heed to your body" (I Corinthians 3:16).

Important Questions

What do you think about this picture of ill health and disease in the body? Do you think it is normal? Do you think it is totally due to living in a fallen world and something we just have to put up with? Does it disturb you? Do you think it is God's ideal? Is it God's fault we get sick? Can we blame it on him? Is it the devil's fault? Is the devil holding your fork? What is wrong? Is this the promised abundant life Jesus died to give? If it is, we should be praying that everyone get cancer.

Heaven forbid! So, what is missing? Clearly, something is. Whatever is missing does matter.

You Don't Need to Get Sick in Order to Die

A woman came up to me after a seminar and said, "Lilli, how am I ever going to die if I never get sick?" She was really concerned about that! What she did not know is that sickness was never God's plan. God's plan is for each one of us to be fully "used up" before we just go to sleep and go home to be with the Lord.

You Might Say, "Isn't Suffering a Part of the Cross We Bear in the Christian Life?"

There are many forms of suffering from living in this fallen world. **However, the suffering we are addressing in this book is suffering as a result of our lifestyle choices, not suffering for the cause of Christ.** *It does not come out of the blue. The diseases we are experiencing in America and in the Christian community are from what we are eating and drinking, primarily.* God wants us well.

Heart disease, cancer, arthritis, asthma, diabetes, osteoporosis, and fibromyalgia are all degenerative diseases, and they are directly attributable to what we put into our bodies. *We do suffer if we have them,* ***but we are not suffering for the cause of Christ,*** so let's be clear about that. Let's connect those dots. Those diseases are coming from what we are not giving our bodies according to God's nutritional design or from what we are putting in our bodies—that is what makes us sick.

Does God Have a Perspective?

There are voices clamoring all around us with confusing messages. When it comes to the subject of health, everyone seems to have an opinion. For example, at every checkout counter, someone is telling you how to take charge of your health. You can hear all kinds of buzz on the Internet, and it can be very conflicting and confusing. We do not need to be gullible. I think it is helpful to ask, "Who is behind the information I am hearing or reading?" Usually *"they say"* people have their own agenda. But what is God's perspective? Do their suggestions line up with God's Word and will? After all, His perspective is the only one that really matters. He is our Father, nutritionist, and designer, and He knows best. Remember the television show back in the 50s, *Father Knows Best?* Well, He really does! Do the ***"they say"*** people really know you?

Many well-meaning people say, "God is sovereign and it is up to God whether I live or die. After all He says He has numbered our days." Sounds spiritual, doesn't it? But God commands *us* to choose life. And He has given us instructions on how to go about that. He instructs us with His eye upon us—He cares. He tells us to eat the right kinds of foods and think the right kinds of thoughts so that our body can be the healer. That's how He designed your body—to be the healer and keep you strong. Why? So that you may live a long, full, and satisfied life and not experience *long, lingering, and painful illnesses* that are a part of the curse. Choose life (in what you eat, what you think, and in what you say) that you and your descendants may live (Deuteronomy 30:19). Don't forget that it is not just about you. How you are caring for your bloodstream and cells gets passed down to your grandchildren and bloodline. We are to pass down an inheritance to our children and grandchildren. What kind of inheritance of physical health are you passing down? Do you have an uncle who, in his eighties, proudly says, "I can eat whatever I want and I'm not sick?" Yet his grandson is dying of cancer, which is the number one cause of death in children under the age of thirteen (next to accidents). How do you think that happens? It happens from the toxic and nutritionally deficient gene pool that is being passed down.

When a pastor asks those who need physical healing in his congregation to stand, and two-thirds of the congregation stands, ***something is missing.***

We are fervently and diligently praying for loved ones and friends who are ill. This is good. I am not inferring that we shouldn't pray, *but is prayer enough?*

When our loved ones and friends are diagnosed, they are immediately put on everyone's prayer list. But how many are being healed?

And how many are living a long and healthy life as a result of prayer alone? Statistics show that *only a small percentage* get some form of healing for the long haul. A small percentage is not nearly enough. Let's be aware that there are many cultures today that eat *God's groceries,* and they aren't sick. In fact, they don't have prayer lines at all. Most of these people are living well beyond one hundred. For those in the Christian community who do get some form of healing, *their sickness returns within six months if they have not addressed the cause of their sickness.* True healing encompasses body, mind, and spirit. I believe if we cure an illness, yet do not address the emotional, spiritual, and dietary issues that surround that ailment, it will only be manifested again somewhere in the body sooner than later.

People are not getting sick due to prayer deficiency; they are getting sick due to cellular nutritional deficiency and toxicity. Our sixty to one hundred trillion cells are made up of proper organic vitamins (not synthetic), minerals, and proper organic amino acids. Our cells, on the other hand, are being bombarded by hundreds of toxic foods, chemicals, herbicides, pesticides, and just about everything that wasn't here a hundred years ago. Let's connect those dots. This is something we do have control over, to some degree.

But what if the Christian community were being taught how to prevent disease in the first place? Do you think we could then be a healthy, shining light to a sick world? How would your church look if your congregation was predominantly physically healthy and not on a long list of medicines? I have found that it is difficult for an unbeliever to hear and receive the gospel from a sick or obese believer. I have worked the college campuses across the nation in evangelism with Cru (formerly Campus Crusade for Christ). I have heard the remarks of unbelievers pertaining to the hypocrisy they perceive. Paul says, "I bring my body into subjection, lest when I have preached to others, I be considered or viewed as a counterfeit" (1 Corinthians 9:27). Remember, it is God who looks at the heart; man tends to look at the outward appearance. We need to walk and live in wisdom with that sensitivity and let our lives reflect the beauty of the Lord in body, soul, and spirit. We then could be contagious in a beautiful way to the sick world.

To know how to live out our days well, happy, fulfilled, and with strength for the battles ahead, we need this wisdom and information from God's Word. We can prevent and heal the diseases that are killing us in our nation if we use the correct weapons God has provided for healing and preventing disease. **Eating properly as if our life depends on it is a mighty spiritual weapon given to us by God against sickness and disease.** Think about all the lives that could be spared! Prayer is only one facet. Confessing that by God's stripes we are healed is but another facet. The physical body will need more unless we are only looking for a quick and temporary "fix" and then needing *another miracle after miracle after miracle.*

Think of all the time and energy that is spent in the body of Christ on prayer for healing of the physical body. Perhaps that energy and precious time could be directed to other significant subjects, like teaching what the Bible has to say about how to walk in health!

What Are the Main Weapons God Has Given Us to Fight Off Disease?

Praise God for prayer; we should always pray without ceasing, but what we are lacking is the *knowledge* of how to walk in health and not get sick in the first place. God's people are perishing for lack of truth in this arena; it is not for lack of prayer or faith. Yet those are the main weapons believers use to fight off sickness and disease.

The subjects of prayer and having faith are exceedingly dominant in the body of Christ. Prayer is a huge component of the Christian life. We desperately need prayer. We are thankful for it. But the physical body does not run on prayer and faith alone. Our physical body has not yet been redeemed. And we are not being taught the practical aspects of living long and well while we are on planet Earth. The human body still runs on physical laws that God set in place from the beginning of time. When we get to heaven, we won't need the physical laws, but we do need them now for living out our number of days well and strong and for carrying out our missions. In fact, we need to be eating as if our life depends on it. ***Because it does.***

For More Clarification, Let's Consider Some of the Systems in Our Physical Body That Need Something More Than <u>Just</u> Prayer

These are some of the systems your doctor will want checked during your annual physical.

Does your body have any of the following?

1) the respiratory system . . . health of the lungs
2) the nervous system
3) the digestive system
4) the excretory system
5) the endocrine system
6) the skeletal and muscular systems
7) the circulatory system
8) the lymphatic system
9) the optic nerves
10) the liver
11) the heart

Are You Giving Your Body Systems More Than Prayer for Functioning Optimally?

Many, if not most, adult believers are already on a long list of medicines for each of the above systems. Yet medicines will not promote health and long life on the cellular level, thus we are living a lie. Not only that, every medicine has bizarre, toxic side effects that create even more illness. Is that God's ideal plan? Or does He have something better in mind? His neutraceuticals have no toxic side effects . . . **only benefits.**

The following is a list of many popular medications which Americans tend to live on without much thought. For so many, these are a daily staple.

Would the following list be a "*trick*" or a "*treat*"?

Maalox
Aluminum hydroxide causes gastrointestinal problems and Alz-

heimer's. Gastrointestinal problems can only be healed by eating the foods that are good for you, not by a medicine that is poisoning you.

Tylenol and "baby" aspirin

They may seem harmless, but they also cause bleeding of the stomach or ulcers. There are much healthier ways to thin our blood.

Statin drugs

This class of drugs can cause loss of memory, muscle strength, and sexual vitality along with erectile dysfunction.

Prozac

According to my understanding, every school, shopping center, and church that has been blown up or shot up was done by someone on antidepressants, Ritalin, or something similar. Some of the side effects of antidepressants are suicide or murder. God is not the author of death and murder. He has a much better way to deal with anxiety and depression.

Metformin

Metformin destroys vitamin B12 (a very important vitamin). Diabetes is caused by poor nutrition and corrected by *proper* nutrition.

Vioxx

Forty thousand people died of a heart attack from this drug before they pulled it. The manufacturer, Merck and Company, knew all along it was not safe yet would not pull it off the market until the deaths of all those people.

Nexium or Prilosec

Doctors don't use these medications themselves, but they prescribe them for their patients. They can cause headaches, dizziness, depression, nausea, pain in the upper abdomen, and many allergic reactions. Nexium and Prilosec are antacids and block the assimilation of proper acid in the stomach for digesting calcium and other nutrients. These are never to be taken longer than fourteen days, yet most who are taking these are uninformed. Many who take them have been living on them for years.

NSAIDs

These are non-steroidal anti-inflammatory drugs like Motrin, Aleve, and ibuprofen, which are sold over the counter. The prescription forms like Celebrex, Voltaren, etc. kill over sixteen thousand people each year from intestinal hemorrhaging alone. And remember, they also foster blood clots. Over one hundred thousand victims a year suffer congestive heart failure from these medications, while who knows how many hip and knee replacements, because of the known cartilage destruction caused by these FDA-approved drugs.

When I pray for someone who has congestive heart failure, I will ask the person if they have been on NSAIDs. I also will offer to give them information on what foods are causing their disease but only if they are open.

Chemotherapy

Is this the answer for cancer? Chemo is a poison and kills healthy cells. In fact, it sometimes kills people faster than the disease itself. It does not sustain a long and healthy life.

Viagra

Listen closely to all the ads you've heard for this drug. "Ask your doctor if you are healthy enough for sexual activity." What does that tell you? Some side effects of Viagra include headaches, *heart attacks,* loss of hearing, tinnitus, eye pain, eye hemorrhage, cataracts, etc. Don't you think there is a better way? We carry many natural products that work wonders with this concern and also provide other benefits to every cell of the body. Despite the side effects, many men in our nation still order this toxic drug.

If you are taking any of the above, know there is a much better way to live your life . . . there are far superior solutions and answers.

We can pray, but if we don't give the physical systems of the body what they need nutritionally, they will not function well. We can't trick nature. The physical human body is designed to function on proper nutrients like vitamins, minerals, and amino acids. That is it. Every medication (from baby aspirin to chemo) has toxic side effects and blocks the flow of true healing. This inevitably leads to your need for more and more pharmaceuticals. We can't just pray or medicate it away. That can be akin to witchcraft. Most are eating the standard American diet, which is outrageous. And then we pray over our symptoms for healing! Who are we kidding? *God help us!*

It's a physical law as long as we are on this earth. You might say something I have heard many times from different people who have come across my path like "Don't give me that law; I am not under the law!" The truth is, there is only one way to heaven, and that is through faith in Jesus Christ. We are not teaching biblical laws for salvation, but that it may go well with you while you are on the earth. **And it is not going well for far too many of us.** If you don't think you are under a law, try driving on the freeways. Try sticking your finger in an electrical socket. You are under laws as long as you are alive on the earth.

In Matthew, Jesus told us that the physical laws are with us until the end of the age and that includes how to take care of our bodies (temples). It is not selfish or sinful to take proper care of your body. You have only been given one body, and God commands us to take care of it. As 1 Corinthians 6:19 so clearly states, "Know ye not that your body is the temple of the Holy Spirit, so take heed to how you care for it." Is that a command or a suggestion? You wouldn't put junk all over the altar at your church, so we shouldn't be putting junk into our bodies and then asking everyone to pray for us when we're sick. I don't mean to sound insensitive, but sometimes, we just need a good healthy dose of truth and tough love. Are you neglecting the care of your physical body? Then you do not love your body, which God says is sacred.

If someone asks you to pray for their healing, ask them also to show you a list of everything they have eaten in the last week. I am not kidding! God's first command was a grocery list that prevents and heals all of the diseases that are killing us. It is God's original health plan mandate. That doesn't sound very spiritual, but God knew that a well-functioning mind and body were necessary to be able to pray, teach the Word, pastor a church, or function in an end-time army!

Want some good news? Here is a list of the some of the benefits you can experience when you give the physical body God's perfect grocery list!

1) Your body is able to reproduce a new liver in just six months.
2) Your body cells are able to reproduce and become totally new in just eleven months.
3) Every ounce of bone in your body can become totally new in just two years.
4) Every blood cell can rejuvenate and become new in just eleven months.
5) We make about sixty million cells every minute of every day.
6) The body replaces itself totally every seven years. It will replace itself healthily depending upon what you're feeding it on all levels.

How? Only when we give the physical body the nutrients God intended. This is the greater and better miracle.

There are two kinds of miracles in the Bible:

1) Dounamis
2) Exhousias

These two very noteworthy miracles in the Bible are different: Dounamis is the miraculous healing and the laying on of hands. Exhousias is the understanding of God's principles for any subject, then obeying, applying, and walking in those principles, which produces a huge lifestyle miracle. It is my opinion that Exhousias is the greater miracle. When we are walking in the Exhouias miracle, we are less likely to need the instantaneous laying on of hands miracle.

Let's picture two doors. For the sake of illustration, which do you choose?

Miracles or blessings?

Both have a function, but blessings are preferable.

It's time for all of us to grow up in new ways!

Being instantaneously healed is one thing; it is the miracle of Dounamis. It is a blessing. However, *may I note that it is for the crisis intervention?* Walking in health is a far greater miracle; it is the miracle of Exhousiasis. You simply cannot live and function on a miracle a day. It was never God's plan to rescue His children out of their health crisis every minute of every day (or even weekly) with an instantaneous miracle. He admonishes us to grow up.

I once was accused of having a "health theology!" What is the alternative? What kind of theology would you want—a sickness, disease, and death theology? That would not be God's theology. The Bible is a book of health and long life. Practically every chapter in the Bible is a chapter about health and how to live a long and full life. However, far too many in the Christian community are living with long, lingering, and painful illnesses. This is profoundly sad and so unnecessary since God has redeemed us from the curse. These diseases are not part of His plan. He is not the author of sickness and disease.

Dr. Gary Null has expressed the seriousness of our health crisis better than anyone. He said, *"If there were a plane crash, where a few hundred people die, it would make the front page of the news for days. But when a million people die in our nation of heart disease or a half million die of cancer, you'd think there would be more of an outcry. It's the equivalent of a jumbo jet full of people crashing every single hour of every single day of every single month for an entire year—year after year after year."*

Where is the Outcry? Have We Just Accepted This as Being Part of a Fallen World?

Most people who have had heart attacks and strokes were not aware they had a problem, and many do not even make it to the hospital. Many times, the first symptom is a massive coronary. Tim Russert, the American television journalist who died suddenly at age fifty-eight, was an example, yet he had the best of medical care, which could not save him. Was he on an eating program for prevention? **People don't know they have cancer either, as cancer can reside in the body for**

seven years before it can be diagnosed or detected.

What about "Early Detection?"

I thank God for early detection and I also thank God for His plan of prevention, which I believe is preferable.

I hear people say, "Oh, thank God for early detection." But what if these people had known how to prevent? Sadly, most don't. *Most believers do not have a clue that the* **very foods they are eating are making their physical body sick**—most think it is the devil making them sick. The reality is, the devil does not need to make us sick. We are making ourselves sick. Does that shock you?

Even in our most brilliantly educated circles, most have never heard this message and are dying of disease prematurely. There are thousands of people in our churches who have cancer and don't even know it. It will be just a matter of time before they get the diagnosis. Everyone around them is in shock and they are put on the prayer lists. Is this enough? Isn't it time to walk in wisdom and *begin training people* in what they eat and don't eat to prevent these diseases? *I, for one, have dedicated my life to equipping the Body of Christ in this subject. It is my opinion that next to the message of salvation, nothing is more important.* God's connection with being healthy is the very food we eat and the very thoughts we think. In Exodus 15:26, He says, "*If you will obey me and keep my statutes and do what I say, I will be your health.*" Does this sound conditional to you? *Being healthy is offered with a condition. If* we listen, *if* we obey, *He will be our health.* He then immediately begins to address blessing their food and water.

Several years ago, I spoke in a wonderful church in Dallas. When the pastor introduced me to his congregation, he said, "What this lady has to say is just as important as any sermon I could ever deliver." Now that's a pastor after my own heart! It set the stage for me to deliver an anointed message and for his congregation to hear with anointed ears and hearts! Because of their shepherd's endorsement of me, it set the stage for them to be able to hear and receive. This is the kind of environment we need in all churches if we are going to be a strong, healthy army and if we are going to be a shining example for the world to see.

There is no condemnation here, but it is very difficult to witness to an unbeliever if you are overweight and unhealthy, as so many believers unfortunately are. Very simply, it is not appealing. Man does still look on the outward appearance. It is God who looks at the heart of man, but even His first priority above everything is that we be in balance and in health: body, soul, and spirit (3 John 1:2). We are not just soul and spirit, but rather body, soul, and spirit.

Aren't These Diseases Just Part of Getting Older?

Do you ever hear remarks like, "I guess I'm just getting older"? I hear this from forty- and fifty-year-olds. Growing older has nothing to do with it! Baby boomers are now becoming "senior boomers!" But many are blaming their diseases on getting older. We hear people refer to their "senior moments." Instead, they should aptly say, "My brain is not functioning well due to oxygen deprivation, which is due to clogged arteries from the foods I have been eating." *Not from old age. There are many cultures today* that do not have any of the diseases that are killing us, and they are living well beyond one hundred. The only difference is their lifestyle and the food they eat. Who is responsible for your health? Is it your doctor, your spouse, your pastor, or is the devil controlling your health? Each one of us must take responsibility for our own health.

You Can Read All about the Lifestyle Differences in the Chapter Entitled "Other Cultures"

Some like to blame their sickness on the devil. Is he the one holding your fork? I suppose the devil could put sickness on you, *but he doesn't need to.* Sometimes these same people are expending tremendous energy rebuking the devil in long healing services, but they are not addressing the cause. I once heard a well-meaning pastor say, "The devil didn't like my ministry so he put this cancer on me." The devil can do a lot of damage on Earth, but he doesn't put the top killer diseases on us without our choosing to ignore God's dietary instructions. I guess he could, but he doesn't need to. **Did the devil cook your breakfast or drive you to the drive-through this morning?**

If you have cancer, you have not been healthy for a long time. ***Cancer does not happen to healthy people.*** We are killing ourselves and literally committing suicide with our own forks and lifestyle choices. You may take chemo, but chemo will not make you healthy.

The blame game goes all the way back to the garden—"the devil tricked me." God has given us the power of choice. Choose life; choose wisdom for a long and healthy life. It is possible and noteworthy, and it is important. Let other responsibilities take a backseat and make your health a priority. You are the only one responsible for your own health. Each of us must take charge of our own health. Everything else you are doing in your ministry or life should be secondary. It's called ordering your private world God's way. Women are notorious for taking great care of everyone else's health in the family and neglecting their own. I see many young moms who are in adrenal exhaustion. They have taken great care of everyone else in the family but have neglected their own health and are burning out. But even adrenals can be replenished with proper nutrients.

CHAPTER 1

Why the Subject of Health Is More Important Today Than Ever Before

Where Is the Outcry?

Next to our eternal salvation, nothing is more important than the health of our body.

If you were asked, "What is the primary interest of people around the world?" what would your answer be? Would you answer love, sex, money, popularity, or fame? All of those sound wonderful. But without your health and wellbeing, you cannot enjoy any of them.

In a multi-year research study carried out by the University of Chicago, the YMCA, and the Association of Adult Education, researchers found that the number one interest of Americans is their health. Why? Nothing can be enjoyed in life if you don't have your health. Yet most, including well-educated teachers, doctors, lawyers, etc., do not know how to take charge of their own health. Why? It is a subject that has *NOT* been emphasized.

How many sermons have you heard on God's delicious and healthy grocery list? This book is devoted to educating believers about nutrition from the latest in cutting-edge science as well as from a *biblical perspective*. And it is important that we begin to educate the body of Christ on how to walk in health in their physical bodies. The answers go way back to the beginning in the Word. They are now being confirmed by medical science. **Science is always having to catch up with God's Word.**

In my private health practice and ministry, I have yet to see one believer who was eating a diet of prevention, and that is out of the thousands who have sought my counsel. They had all been minding their own business, going about their day with their morning quiet time, reading the Word, studying, and praying, but they were also eating the diet of Egypt *(the world's diet)*. And many come to see me because they are suffering the *diseases* of Egypt. Because they are suffering in their health, they begin to assume this is what they must endure to share in Christ's suffering. Suffering for Christ's sake occurs when we are persecuted because we are believers, and we are light in a very dark and fallen world. The light exposes the darkness. But sickness and degenerative disease is a result of our own lifestyle choices, not for the cause of Christ.

If you have ever had cancer or heart disease, you would give everything you had to have your health back. It saddens me that most do not know how to prevent cancer in the first place. Many think that it has come through genetics, or they just seem to "catch it." Genetics accounts for about 20 percent of the equation. The other 80 percent amounts to our own lifestyle choices. We also inherit our parent's eating habits and tastes.

This subject is more important today than ever before in history. Ironically, we are less healthy today than our presidents were 250 years ago. This is despite the trillions of dollars we've spent looking for a cure. In fact, we are no further along than when President Nixon declared the "War on Cancer" in 1971. The cure will never be found in a test tube of chemicals. So run for your own health, not for more medical research. We know the answer to preventing and curing cancer and all other degenerative diseases. God gave us the answer four thousand years ago, but we have not been taught.

Why Is This Important?

Because we are very, very sick as a nation, and the body of Christ may be sicker than the world. Why is this? Many are eating mindlessly and what we don't know is hurting us. Many are presuming they can eat whatever they want since they are no longer under a law for salvation. We should be eating as if our life depends upon it. Most are eating as if their food choices don't matter. I can't think of any other area of our lives where we are so reckless and irresponsible. Would we be this nonchalant with our finances, our checkbooks, or the care of our vehicles?

Why Is This Important?

God has given us a mandate to steward the temple we have been given, but we are not being educated and equipped to do it. Maybe we don't really think it is possible in today's world. Most in the Christian community do not even know that the foods they are eating are making them sick. Most believe they can eat anything and be fine as long as they pray over it. How is that theology working for the body of Christ? We need to begin to connect some dots. I have heard many say they did not know God had anything to say about what we eat.

I once had a missionary tell me she did not need this message, that she ran on the Spirit. This sounds very good and spiritual, but what she was not acknowledging is that the Spirit is the same yesterday, today, and forever. The Holy Spirit is the One who gave us the guidelines for the physical part of our body. That inspired Holy Spirit has not changed. Soon after she made that pronouncement, she was brought home from the mission field with adrenal exhaustion. We can't fool the system God gave us. We can't play tricks with His instructions and act as if they do not exist. He gave us guidelines for the body, the soul, and the spirit, and all three must be respectively nourished. They are all needed now while we are on Earth.

When we get to heaven, we won't need dietary laws or even the law of gravity, but we do need them now for walking in blessing and not harm. *We are not teaching dietary laws for salvation; we share them so that it may go well with you NOW on the earth.* Have you heard a lot of teaching on this subject? We have lives to live here and assignments to complete. We have eighty to one hundred trillion cells in our bodies. These cells run on nutrients like amino acids, vitamins, and minerals—not Maalox, Metformin, Tylenol, chemotherapy, Nexium (the "purple pill"), or Viagra. We have the optic nerve, the heart muscle, the pancreas, the lungs, bowels, kidneys, and a liver. **Every organ and every cell runs on physical laws.** When one organ begins to break down, it will affect the rest of the body. Just as our automobiles are finely tuned, so are our bodies. We don't generally just pray over our cars when they don't have gas or oil; it's a no-brainer to put in the necessary ingredients that make them run properly. Our cars come with a manufacturer's manual. If the gas tank is empty, we don't just stuff a banana in the gas tank; the car is not made to run on bananas. We just simply fill up the gas tank. Our cars run well with the proper kind of fuel. *Likewise, our body came into this world with its own unique owner's manual.* First Corinthians 6:19: "Know ye not that your body is the temple of the Holy Spirit. You are not your own." We are admonished not to defile our bodies. There are many Christians who would never think of committing murder, adultery or getting drunk, yet they consume 150 pounds of sugar annually. *And Americans eat one million dead animals an hour!* That hardly lines up with God's proven program of prevention. In the chapter "Foods That Heal," we list the fresh fruits and vegetables that are needed for prevention. There are no antioxidants in sugar or animals to prevent cancer, for example.

Most believers are constantly eating foods that God said would be an abomination (abomination means you will be sick). Was this just for the Old Testament? In Leviticus 11, He addresses the food group we call meat and dairy and says, *for all the generations to come,* do not eat certain animals. Would for all the generations to come be just for the Old Testament or for the nation of Israel? In Romans 12, we are admonished to present our bodies as a living sacrifice to Him. He admonishes us that if we don't bring our bodies in subjection, we may be counted as a counterfeit or a castaway (1 Corinthians 9:27). That admonition sounds serious!

There is a plethora of confusing information being distributed on this topic. What is God's perspective? Thousands of books have been written on health, but few are targeting the root cause of our sickness. And few are addressing health from a biblical perspective. We don't need the world to tell us how to take charge of these temples. Our Father gave us instructions four thousand years ago.

The Christian community is sadly ignorant of how to care for the human body according to God's design.

After I had just finished speaking on this topic at a church in Dallas, a woman came up to me afterwards and said, "Lilli, this subject needs to precede all other topics on *any seminar platform.*" I agree. And I believe this is about to happen. It *must*, if we are going to live well, fulfill our callings, and not die prematurely. Sickness is a thief, not a blessing. There are far too many sick believers who blame it on the fallen world or on the devil.

Why Is This Subject So Important to Emphasize As Never Before?

Between the medicines they take and the doctors they see, most Americans are preoccupied with their illnesses. *This is bondage.* As a point of illustration, I often hear this fact borne out when I'm having my nails done at the salon. Very often, women are sharing and empathizing with each other about their latest diagnosis, favorite oncologist, and all the different medical tests they are undergoing. These are women of all ages, mind you, not just the elderly. Medicine, hospitals, and Big Pharma have become daily household words. We are being robbed in the workplace and the home. We are being robbed of quality of life and productivity. We are being robbed of our peaceful family relationships *because of ill health.*

Yet we are creatures of purpose and destiny—not just chance. When you are sick and tired, your ministry is hindered. You don't feel very spiritual or loving or patient. You call your prayer committee and ask them to pray for healing. Even if God heals you, the healing usually will not remain if the cause of the physical problem is not addressed. Jesus said to the woman at the well, "I forgive you, now go and sin no more." He put the responsibility for her continued deliverance and freedom back on her for her lifestyle choices. He is still doing that today. No one can take charge of your health for you.

People look forward to going on a luxurious cruise, a trip abroad, or even retirement. But do they feel well? Can you imagine being able to enjoy any of those activities if you don't feel well? To a man or woman suffering with cancer, happiness would be a healthy body—not a million dollars or a cruise. A person with cancer would give anything to have his health back. The average cancer patient spends $50,000 on his disease in his lifetime.

Why Is This Important?

People are going to their doctors, plopping their symptoms down, and saying, "I want my health back. I will pay you whatever you ask, Doctor, if you will just give me my health back." But the doctor can't give it. True health is not found in a test tube, a prescription drug, or an organ being removed or transplanted. Sometimes, these things are needed, but they do not offer quality of health for the long haul. The textbooks for medical doctors are written by the pharmaceutical companies. Doctors are trained in prescription drugs and surgery, not in how to heal the body. They are not educated in nutrition. They are sadly dying early of all the diseases we are teaching people to avoid because they typically do not have this knowledge.

My own OB/Gyn doctor was an excellent physician at Dallas Baylor Hospital. Whereas I desperately needed him to deliver my babies, I did not need him to tell me how to take charge of my health. He died of colon cancer, and his beautiful wife died of breast cancer. He did not think what he ate yesterday could make a difference in his health today. The subject of eating healthily was like Greek to him. He, like so many excellent physicians, did not understand the revelatory connection between illness and the foods we eat.

This subject is vitally important. While other subjects are being highly emphasized, this one has been tragically neglected. We don't need to have our heads in the sand. This message is pretty simple, really, and life changing.

One of the first commands God gave us was a grocery list of what to eat. In Genesis 1:29 and 30, He addresses the foods we are to eat *for all the generations to come* to live a long and prosperous life. This subject is one of His top priorities. In 3 John 2 He says, "Above everything else in the whole world, I want you to prosper and be healthy as your soul prospers." With the status of our health as it is, I believe we need to take a fresh look at one of God's top priorities, which we have neglected. There will be no change unless our souls, minds, and hearts are renewed with the truth. Genesis 1:29 and 30 was His original health plan mandate, and it still is today. Many cultures are adhering to His original health plan and diet and they have practically zero statistics of disease. Maybe we better take a fresh look.

CHAPTER 2

The Status of the American Population Where Health Is Concerned

According to the World Health Organization and the American Medical Association, *America is in the worst chronic epidemic of degenerative diseases known to mankind.* As a Christian nation, we lead the world in degenerative diseases. It is no longer a germ attacking us from the outside for which we can be immunized; these are the diseases that are coming from what we are putting in our bodies. We are decaying from within. These are diseases for which we can't blame the devil. We rank 150th in world health.

What Is Happening in Our World Where Health Is Concerned?

Many may not know that heart disease is one of the leading causes of death in the U.S. and we have over a million people a year *who die from preventable heart disease.*

These chronic degenerative diseases are among the leading cause of death and disability in the United States and, of course, that includes the Christian community. Degenerative diseases cause seven out of ten deaths each year. Heart disease, cancer, and strokes alone cause more than 50 percent of all deaths each year. Please note that people who are diagnosed with cancer, cardiovascular issues, or diabetes, just to name a few, have not been healthy for a long time. It takes about seven years of disease being resident before a diagnosis can be made. *Prevention is far superior to early detection . . . and these diseases are preventable.*

The United States is number one in the world! Right?

But not so fast . . . we rank number one in many areas, but poorly in the following:

- Heart disease
- Cancer
- Diabetes
- Alzheimer's
- Obesity

Are these the diseases of the elderly? No. Do we inherit these diseases? Again, no. We can attribute 20 percent to genetics and then a whopping 80 percent to lifestyle choices. There are many cultures today that do not have any of these diseases. There are cultures living beyond one hundred. They are not sick. Why? They are eating the Mediterranean or Bible diet. They do not claim to be Christians. We discuss more specifics about other healthy cultures in a later chapter.

According to *National Vital Statistics Reports* (Vol. 57, No. 14), 2,426,264 Americans died in 2006. It reports the ten leading causes of death in the United States as follows:

Heart Disease 724,859
Cancer 541,532
Stroke 158,448
COPD 112,584
Accidents 97,835
Pneumonia/Influenza 91,871
Diabetes 64,751

Suicide. 30,575
Kidney Disease 26,182
Liver Disease & Cirrhosis. 25,192

Seven out of the ten leading causes of death in the United States have been linked directly to our diet. *Three out of four in the obituary columns* in the newspapers are dying from these same preventable degenerative diseases. The Father is calling all of us to take note, pay attention, and show up with hungry and thirsty hearts and ears to hear the truth on this topic. While we are on the earth, we are still body, soul, and spirit. Are you giving each of those parts the nourishment intended by your loving Father? If you are neglecting the body, you will not live out the number of your days that God's best offers you. *It doesn't matter if you are Billy Graham, Oswald Chambers, or Dwight L. Moody, you can be studying and confessing the word all day long and you may be having a fruitful ministry to some extent, but if your pantries are filled with the world's dainties instead of God's groceries, your life and ministry will be shortened.* And not by the devil or because God just wanted to take you home early: it will be shortened because you have not had ears to hear, so you are suffering in your body. The apostle Paul is calling to us and saying, "Oh, foolish believers, who has bewitched you?" God offers a better way. His nutrients only bring life, and that is their only side effect.

Besides accidents, which kill less than one hundred thousand Americans each year, the vast majority of deaths are caused by poor diet and lifestyle choices. We are literally committing suicide with our own spoons and forks. If every American made a simple change in their diet and lifestyle, the list above would greatly diminish. We can't change everything overnight, but I say you attack this subject like a worm attacks an apple, one bite at a time! Even small changes can make a big difference, like adding twenty-nine years to your life! Now that's a valuable concept!

Drug-related Deaths in Our Nation

They are staggering. Drug-related death is actually the number one cause of death in our nation even exceeding the diseases that are killing us.

The *Physician's Desk Reference* contains over three thousand pages of adverse reactions—including death—that may result in patients who are taking these drugs.

Often, a patient may enter the hospital with symptoms of heart disease and actually die of pneumonia. They didn't have pneumonia until they entered the hospital. However, the medication given to that patient may cause the elimination organs to become so clogged that the lungs fill up with fluid and drown the patient. Have you noticed the upward trend in deaths caused by pneumonia? As believers begin to rely more and more on drugs instead of God's sensible nutrients, these numbers will continue to rise. Every drug has a dangerously toxic side effect. Yet most trust our doctors to know best and mindlessly take the purple pill or the medicine to sleep or whatever. Most do not even hear the horrible side effects mentioned on television ads. Many times, the side effects are death while we think we are taking something for our health. Talk about an upside-down world! Paul addressed the Galatians and said, "Oh foolish Galatians, who has bewitched you?" We have been bewitched by Big Pharma, which is sorcery. Medicine has its place, but never for the long haul. It should be used only for a crisis. Twenty percent of medicine is good—if you are having a baby, have an eye socked out, need surgery, or tests run. But the other 80 percent fails miserably. It does not produce a long, healthy life. At best, it can prolong some years, but not the quality of health. The cultures where the people are living healthily beyond the age of one hundred are not on medicines.

Even the American Medical Association's own medical journal admits that over 106,000 Americans die each year from reactions to prescription drugs. Dr. C. Everett Koop, the former US surgeon general, confirmed that over two million people are hospitalized from the side effects as well.

What Are Iatrogenic Deaths?

According to Webster's Dictionary, iatrogenic death is defined as "induced unintentionally by the medical treatment of a physician." This category would also include mistakes made in surgery and hospital care by doctors and nurses. Iatrogenic deaths are estimated to be at least 783,936 per year, **placing it as the number one cause of death in America.**

According to Dr. Gary Null in his book entitled *Death by Medicine,* 50,000 people die from malnutrition each year after being in a hospital. They weren't malnourished before they went into the hospital, but after being on hospital food and under dietetic care, they died. How many people died of infections they did not have until they went into the hospital? In 2013 alone, 107,000 died from infections in hospitals. How about unnecessary medical procedures? Dr. Null says an estimated 7.5 million unnecessary medical and surgical procedures are performed each year. These were unnecessary surgeries. How many medical procedures are unnecessary? How many people get medicines they shouldn't have because of this? How many people get tests they don't need so that the doctor is protected in case there is a lawsuit? The number one cause of *death* in America is from medicine (iatrogenic deaths). This exceeds even the degenerative deaths. Minimally, 783,936 dead—and that's just a conservative figure Null's team came up with. More practically, 1 million. The leading cause of *injuries in America is medicine*; almost 11 million injured. So what you have is 11 million injured and 783,936 dead. Let's consider that over a ten-year period. You have 8 million dead Americans and 190 million injuries—that's quite a staggering cost. The projected statistic of 7.8 million iatrogenic deaths is more than all the casualties from wars that America has fought in its entire history. More people are killed by our own medical community each year than terrorists could kill if they blew up the World Trade Center with a jumbo jet every day after day—and who knows for how long.

Dr. Barbara Starfield of the John's Hopkins School of Hygiene and Public Health in Baltimore, Maryland, wrote an article in the July 26, 2000, issue of the *Journal of the American Medical Association* (JAMA), volume 284. She entitled her article "Doctors and Their Drugs Could Be the Number One Cause of Deaths in America."

She listed the following categories of iatrogenic deaths:

- 12,000 deaths/year from unnecessary surgery
- 7,000 deaths/year from medication errors in hospitals
- 20,000 deaths/year from other errors in hospitals
- 80,000 deaths/year from infections in hospitals
- 106,000 deaths/year from non-error, adverse effects of medications

Jesus said He came to give us abundant life. Is this the abundant life?

Deuteronomy says that "God wants to deliver us from these long and lingering illnesses." If we have been redeemed from the curse of the law, why is America and the body of Christ suffering with the following overwhelming statistics? I was in a Bible study the other day, and the subject of cancer came up. Many of the women had already had cancer. One well-meaning woman spoke up and said, "I am tired of people calling it the 'big C.' Christ is the big C. Cancer is nothing." *This sounds real spiritual* but if it is nothing, *why are one in three people (including believers) dying of cancer?* We will answer that question in another chapter. It is not for lack of prayer or faith. There are some things we can't just pray away. But for now, let's take a quick look at these staggering statistics of diseases that are preventable:

- 1 in 2 will die of heart disease.
- 1 in 3 will die of cancer.
- 60 million Americans currently suffer from cardiovascular disease, which includes high blood pressure and strokes.
- 25.8 million Americans are diagnosed with diabetes. That's 8.3 percent of the U.S. population.
- The annual economic cost of diabetes is a staggering $245 billion dollars.
- 43 million suffer from arthritis.
- Osteoporosis affects 28 million Americans. More women die from osteoporosis than breast cancer.

- 42 million people in the world currently have AIDS.
- The number one killer of children under the age of thirteen is cancer (next to accidents).
- 121 million suffer from depression.

Seventy-five percent of US health spending goes to treating these degenerative (preventable) diseases. America spends $2.7 trillion annually on healthcare. That is about $8,500 per person more than any other nation spends. Cancer can cost a patient $50,000 in his or her lifetime. **Incidentally, only four cents of every dollar goes to public health and prevention related activities, sad to say.**

Additionally, over one billion colds occur in the US each year, causing the most common reason for school and work absences. Because approximately 20 percent of the US population attends or works in schools, nearly twenty-two million school days are lost annually due to the common cold alone. The economic and societal impact of colds and the flu is huge. As the most frequent illness among Americans, these viral illnesses annually attack five hundred million times and cost $40 billion in doctor's bills, medication, missed work, and school days, according to a University of Michigan report.

The so-called common cold is aptly named because in a given year, nearly half the US population will catch a cold, and 40 percent will develop influenza. Inevitably, you will hear people say "Everyone is catching this cold" and "There's nothing we could have done to prevent catching this cold." Let's consider the impact that eating sugar has on catching a cold. Do you like to eat sugar? You simply don't catch a cold or anything else if your immune system is healthy. Sugar depletes the immune system of nutrients. Do you eat too much sugar? The average American eats 150 pounds of sugar a year. Just picture thirty 5-pound bags of sugar. We'll discuss this more fully in the chapter entitled "Foods That Kill."

Additionally, tens of millions of people get the flu each year, with some cases resulting in hospitalization or death. The CDC (Centers for Disease Control) estimates 10–20 percent of Americans come down with the flu during flu season, which typically lasts from November to March. The CDC also estimates that in the US alone, more than one hundred thousand people are hospitalized and about thirty-six thousand people die every year from the flu and its resulting complications. Children and the elderly are most susceptible to the damages from the flu.

Nearly everywhere we go, flu shots are being advertised, whether it's the grocery store or drugstore. What is in the flu shot? Every year when the flu season comes around with all of its warnings and advice, why do so many people panic and take in the world's system with its very toxic flu shots? Is it possible that we're afraid because we haven't done our part in keeping healthy so that we don't get the flu in the first place? Is the flu shot the best the medical world has to offer in keeping our immune systems healthy?

What's in the standard flu shot? You should know if you are letting someone inject your bloodstream with something. Remember, the life of the flesh is in the blood. You should know what is going into your body since you are the only one who is responsible for it and your health. God put you in charge of your body, not the medical association.

So, let's take a peek at what is in the shot:

- Egg proteins: including avian contaminant viruses. Many Americans are allergic to eggs, and who wants an avian contaminant virus injected in the blood stream?
- Gelatin, which can cause allergic reactions and anaphylaxis (conditions usually associated with sensitivity to egg or gelatin).
- Polysorbate 80™, which can cause severe allergic reactions, including anaphylaxis. Also associated with infertility.
- Formaldehyde, which is a known carcinogen.
- Triton X100: a strong detergent.
- Sugar.
- Resin, which is known to cause allergic reactions.
- Gentamycin: an antibiotic.
- Thimerosal. Mercury is still in multidose flu shot vials.

Most Americans take the flu shot not knowing or even asking

what's in it. Is this not mindlessly trusting medical doctors, the FDA, and Big Pharma, which can be sorcery? Do you honestly think they can all be trusted? Every single medication has a toxic side effect, and sometimes, the side effect is death. *Is this God's way?* Sometimes, we need medicine for a crisis, but it should never be a daily way of life. That is, if you want to live a long and healthy life. Living daily on meds is basically a lie. It can make you think you are healthy when only the symptoms have been addressed. Medications do not produce health, and they do not address the cause of the sickness. Every medicine has toxic side effects.

According to the 2006 Cochrane Database of Systemic Reviews, "Vaccines for preventing influenza in healthy adults" (a review of forty-eight reports including more than sixty-six thousand adults), "Vaccination of healthy adults only reduced risk of influenza by 6 percent and reduced the number of missed workdays by less than one day (0.16) days. It did not change the number of people needing to go to the hospital or take time off work."

So how do we protect ourselves against disease and other harmful invaders including bacteria and viruses? Is it by antibiotics? Remember, most of these conditions are fungal, which antibiotics don't heal; they only make the condition worse.

God gave us an immune system, which is meant to protect us. But we must give our immune systems the correct raw ingredients to optimally function so they can do just that. How? That would be none other than pure vitamins, minerals, and amino acids—not medicine and processed foods, which clog up the flow of life and health.

Our Trillion Dollar Healthcare Industry Is the Fastest Growing Sector of Our Economy

On January 22, 1971, President Richard Nixon declared total war on cancer in the National Cancer Act of 1971. The National Cancer Institute (NCI) was further charged with coordinating the national cancer program. Many predicted a swift victory. If we could put a man on the moon, surely with all our knowledge and technology, we could whip cancer!

With regard to cancer as a whole, twenty thousand people die of cancer every single day. This translates to eight million deaths every year. Half a million are Americans. Today, one person out of three gets cancer in the course of his or her lifetime. It is not going away, despite all of the trillions of dollars being spent on so-called research. In the 1940s, one in sixteen people developed cancer. In the 1970s, it was one in ten. And now it is one in three. According to the CDC, about 1.66 million new cancer cases are expected to be diagnosed this year in the US.

In the forty-plus years since Nixon engaged America in the battle with cancer, various government and private agencies have spent $200 billion on research with little results. Many critics call this a *"medical Vietnam."* Many say the forty-year-old war on cancer has been a farce. The epidemic is a dream for Big Pharma, and their campaigns to silence cancer cures have been fierce and totally closed-minded, according to the documentary film *Cancer: Forbidden Cures.*

Please understand that cancer is a big business. Contrary to their advertising campaigns, which want you to give for a cure, virtually none of their funding is being spent on preventive cures such as dietary guidelines. Only four cents of every dollar is devoted to lifestyle choices that cause cancer. The typical cancer patient spends $50,000 fighting the disease. Contrast that with the cost of vitamins. Please note, you can budget in $100 to $200 a month toward the best vitamins available, and what do you get? Quality of health and longer life.

In fact, in an article by the American Medical Association in the *New England Journal of Medicine*, Dr. John Bailar and Dr. Elaine M. Smith say, "With respect to cancer as a whole, we have slowly lost ground; we see no reason for optimism about our overall progress. There is no evidence of a recent downward trend; in the clinical sense, we are losing the war against cancer. The main conclusion that we draw is that some forty-plus years of intense effort, focused largely on treatment, must be judged a qualified failure. *A greater focus on preventing cancer through proper eating habits,* changes in lifestyle, and environmental controls may hold much more promise in conquering this disease."

In spite of the trillions being invested in research, as of January 21, 2005, according to the American Cancer Society's latest projections, cancer has displaced heart disease as the leading killer of Americans under the age of eighty-five. The numbers are as stark as death: we are losing the war against cancer and it is not going away. This group predicts that 1,825,400 Americans will be diagnosed with cancer. Sadly, a large percentage will die. Did you know that it is not normal to have cancer, and it doesn't come out of the blue? Healthy people do not get cancer. Cancer is a curse and God's Word states that a causeless curse shall not alight (Proverbs 26:2). Although it is common, it is not normal. God's will and desire is that His children choose life, blessing, and normalcy. But for lack of knowledge and erroneous teaching, God's people (not somebody else's people) are perishing. Americans deserve to know the truth, as do believers.

Lung cancer remains the leading cancer killer, accounting for 31 percent of cancer deaths in men and 27 percent of deaths in women. In men, lung cancer is followed by prostate cancer, then colorectal cancer as the top killers. For women, breast cancer ranks second for mortality, followed by colorectal cancer.

The order of the top three has not changed since the late 1980s, when the number of deaths from lung cancer overtook those of breast cancer in women, and prostate overtook colon and rectal cancer in men.

According to the National Cancer Institute, obese men run a 50 percent greater risk of developing cancer overall. Specifically, that would be cancer of the liver, pancreas, stomach, and esophagus. Obese women face a 70 percent greater cancer risk, particularly cancer of the uterus, kidney, cervix, and pancreas. An article in the *Journal of the American Medical Association* says that one high-risk factor with regard to these particular cancers is the ingestion of too much fat. God told us that four thousand years ago. He told us in Leviticus not to eat the fat for all the generations to come. But we have been taught that is Old Testament law and that now, we are under grace. Isn't it interesting we are not taught that about the moral laws or laws of physics? Jesus said these laws have been given for our good while we are on the earth. In the New Testament in Matthew, He said, "I have not come to destroy the law." When we get to heaven, we won't need these laws, but our bodies have not yet been redeemed. They still run on physical laws.

For greater emphasis, let me say this: if Billy Graham, Oswald Chambers, or Dwight L. Moody were to jump off the Empire State Building, each one of them could confess all the way down that they are a faith-filled Christian, a Word-filled Christian, and that they are not under the law. But they would splatter on the concrete anyway because a law was violated—the law of gravity. These laws are with us until the end of the age, and they are for our own good. It doesn't matter if you know about it or agree with it, it is a law until the end of the age.

About one-third of new cancer cases this year will be due to to-bacco use, another third to poor nutrition, and the final third will be linked to inactivity or obesity. Dr. Harmon Eyre, the Cancer Society's longtime chief medical officer, stated, "We want to send the message: Eat right (most Americans do not have a clue what it means to "eat right"), don't smoke, exercise, maintain normal weight, and see your doctor for annual checkups." Yes, this is prevention! Eating right is very nebulous and confusing for most. That is where the enemy has done everything possible to confuse the message of health with myths and misinformation.

In the history of warfare, it has always been an axiom that if you are losing the battle, change tactics! The main conclusion we draw is that some forty-plus years of intensive effort focused largely on improving treatment must be judged a qualified failure. Our approach to cancer and all degenerative disease needs to be changed.

If medicine and prayer alone were the answer, we would be the healthiest nation in the world. But instead, we are one of the sickest and lead the world in the degenerative diseases. It is becoming more and more apparent that standard medical science is failing when it comes to managing or treating any disease. More people are getting medical treatment, taking more drugs, having more and more diag-nostic testing, and undergoing more surgeries than ever before. *Yet more people are getting sicker than ever before.*

We spent over a trillion dollars on health care in 1997. In fact, the cost of our health care is spiraling so far out of control that the Healthcare Financing Administration predicted that our system would cost sixteen trillion dollars within fifteen years. We spend more on healthcare than any other country. Seventy-five percent of US health spending goes toward treating degenerative diseases. Only four cents out of every dollar is spent on researching prevention. *Prevention must become our focus,* as the current model is not sustainable. We need to begin making small consistent steps which become healthier habits. We cannot depend on our government and agencies. We need to take it upon ourselves to make prevention a personal priority. And this will require a paradigm shift in our thinking.

The Number One Cause of Bankruptcy in Our Nation Is Medical Bills

The Father's heart is to deliver us from long and lingering illnesses (Deuteronomy 28:59). The circumstances in which Americans are dying today are often unnecessarily early, painful, and costly. In fact, Dr. T. Campbell states in his book *The China Study* that **"Americans are paying for their own expensive graves."** It is no wonder, too, that the number one cause of bankruptcy in our nation is due to medical expenses. The Cancer Institute predicts that 50 percent of Americans will have some form of cancer. That's one out of two. We lose over a half million annually to totally preventable cancer. This is so sad and unnecessary.

What about our children? Cancer is the number one killer of children between the ages of four and fourteen, next to accidents. Children are eating all kinds of food that their little bodies cannot digest, i.e., meat, dairy, sugar, and nutritionally void fast foods. Think twice and choose wisely before you give your children Happy Meals. Children under fourteen who have not yet gone through puberty do not have the digestive enzymes to digest meat. That includes hamburgers and hot dogs. Meat is for the mature. Milk is for newborns. That begs the question, why are adults drinking cow's milk? We cover that in a later chapter. What is cancer? Without oversimplification, it is a pancreatic enzyme deficiency. Where do we get enzymes? We get them from raw fresh fruits and vegetables. Notice I said raw. Once a food is cooked over 118 degrees, there are no enzymes, and the pancreas must over-work to produce enzymes for digesting the cooked and devitalized foods. Our Chief Nutritionist gave us a grocery list of foods to eat that have the antioxidants, fiber, and enzymes to prevent cancer and all disease. According to research, only 3 percent of Americans get in the recommended amounts of fresh fruits and vegetables suggested by the food-guide pyramid standard. Isn't it interesting that today you hear a lot about the need for more fiber in the diet to prevent one of our top killers (colon cancer), and you hear a lot about the need for antioxidants to prevent cancer and eye conditions as well? But God's original health plan in Genesis 1:29, 30 is chock-full of the right kind of fiber, antioxidants, and enzymes. The genesis of good health goes all the way back to the beginning . . .

To continue the latest statistics on cancer, forty-three thousand sisters, mothers, and friends will die from breast cancer this year. Let's note the connection between the six million American women who are daily using a synthetic hormone made from the urine of a pregnant mare (premarin). The findings are published in the July 17, 2002, issue of the *Journal of the American Medical Association*. Funded by the Women's Health Initiative, these studies revealed that premarin increased women's risk of stroke by 41 percent, a heart attack by 29 percent, and breast cancer by 24 percent.

Two hundred thousand men will be diagnosed with prostate cancer this year. One-fifth of them will die. It has been said that if you live long enough, you will have prostate problems if you are not doing a program of prevention. If you have to have surgery and radiation and drug therapy, it is only 30 percent effective. Why not try a natural program of cancer prevention foods and selective supplements for the prostate first? You will be amazed at what it can do for you. Research tells us that not smoking, proper nutrition, and exercise can lower risk of one of our top killers by a whopping 66 percent!

The number two disease killer in our nation is cardiovascular disease, and it is taking a new rank.

This would include heart attacks, strokes, and high blood pressure. Our chances of dying of heart disease are now 50 percent. This is not just a man's disease but also the number one killer of women over forty. Heart disease will kill one out of every three Americans. According to the American Heart Association, over sixty million Americans currently suffer from some form of cardiovascular disease, including high blood pressure, stroke, and heart disease. Most of us have been sadly impacted by a loved one or good friend who has died from cardiovascular disease.

More and more knowledge has been uncovered in understanding this disease. There are recent findings that heart disease can be prevented and even reversed by a healthy diet. God told us this in Genesis 1:29, 30. By embracing the information in this book and other like-minded materials, we could collectively defeat the most dangerous killer disease in this country.

One hundred years ago, heart attacks were virtually unknown until the invention of the flour mill. Today the flour will keep until the millennium! With the invention of the flour mill around the turn of the century, the necessary nutrients have been stripped and we have been raped and robbed of the very nutrients that cause our hearts to function properly.

Why is heart disease one of our top killers? Although there are many factors to consider, the B vitamins have been stripped. The vitamin E has been stripped and these, in an organic form, are absolutely essential for protecting the heart.

Consider These Statistics

Last year one million Americans died from some form of cardiovascular disease (CVD). We had 1.5 million heart attacks and 550,000 died. Strokes killed another 150,000. The American Heart Association tells us an amazing sixty-three million Americans have CVD. Seventy-five million have high blood pressure. This is common, but it is not normal. In fact, it is grossly abnormal.

Heart disease and strokes can be a very silent killer. In half of those

550,000 deaths, the first symptom that something was wrong was sudden death. Most people who have a massive coronary heart attack do not even know they have heart disease, and many do not make it to the hospital.

This was the case with Tim Russert, television journalist and lawyer. My understanding is that Tim Russert had just passed a heart stress test. He was being treated with medication that does not heal the body and a breach of one small artery, which burst, caused him to die an untimely death. Is there a better way to keep the arteries clear and flowing? Good nutrition is a start. God gave us the grocery list four thousand years ago, but we have not believed it nor did we want to believe it. If we want to live a long and full life where our latter years are better than our former, we will need to heed. There are no shortcuts, and we can't trick the system by taking all these medications and eating however we want. Every curse has a cause.

But cancer and heart disease are not the only epidemics casting a large shadow over American health. Diabetes has also increased in unprecedented proportions. One out of thirteen Americans now has diabetes and suffers from its complications, including blindness, limb amputation, cardiovascular disease, kidney disease, and various kinds of nervous disorders and premature deaths. Two of the most frightening statistics show that diabetes among people in their thirties has increased 70 percent in the last ten years. Among those in their forties, it has increased 40 percent within a nine-year period. Thirty-four percent of diabetics are not aware of their illness at all. The annual economic cost of diabetes is a staggering $174 billion.

One of the leading causes of death in our nation is our healthcare system itself. One of the most well-regarded voices representing the medical community, the *Journal of the American Medical Association* (JAMA), included a recent article by Barbara Starfield, MD, stating that physician error, medication error, and adverse reactions from drugs or surgery kill 225,400 people per year. As Americans fall victim to any disease, we do hope that our hospitals and doctors will do all that they can to help us. However, both the newspapers and courts are filled with stories and cases that tell us that inadequate care has become very common.

From there, we have allergies, sinus infections, bronchitis, fibromyalgia, migraines, and all of the estrogen-dominant related conditions, i.e., endometriosis, uterine fibroids, PMS, migraines, and infertility.

Antidepressants:
These statistics are depressing!

According to the Centers for Disease Control, twenty-one million Americans are depressed and take antidepressants, which have tragic side effects, including, for example, suicide and murder. Every school and church shooting has been caused by teens that were either on Ritalin or an antidepressant. This also included the young boy who flew a plane into the side of the Bank of America building in Florida. According to the FDA, there were fourteen million prescriptions written in the U.S. for antidepressants in 1992. In 2002, just ten years later, that number had jumped from 14 million to 157 million prescriptions. Eleven million of those were prescribed for children under the age of eighteen, some as young as two to four years old.

There is such a thing as nutrition for brain function, and food is a key factor. Why not consume a lot of essential omega complex with EPA and DHA? There has been a lot of research on the role of essential fatty acids for normalizing brain function; these are the good fats in cold-water fish with fins and scales. They are also in walnuts, flax seeds, and in soy. These also come in organic supplement form as well. This is so vital for depression and bipolar syndrome, and it's helpful for normalizing brain function of all kinds. The only side effect from taking the essential omegas is that they will produce healthy hearts and arteries as well. And who wouldn't want that? That's God's way. Everything He has guided us to do only brings multiple bountiful blessings and positive fruit. Not only can you live longer, but you can *live better while you are living longer!*

Modern medicine can make people live a really long time, but modern medicine cannot necessarily improve the quality of life. The best way to improve and maintain an excellent quality of life as we age is making sure the parts work. We make the parts work by being physically active and by giving the sixty to one hundred trillion cells what they need. These cells and bodies are made up of nutrients in which Americans are deficient. The body was designed to be active. We were not designed to sit all day and stare at the computer and manage emails. One hundred years ago, this was not the case.

To Sum It Up

Despite all of our medicines, treatments, surgeries, and healing lines, Americans do not feel well. We are not healing enough people in the healing lines because the cause and personal responsibility has not been addressed. And as I have suggested, medicine is not the answer, and neither is prayer alone. There simply are some things we can't just pray away. When our cars are malfunctioning, for example, we don't just pray, nor do we cut the wire to the connection that is flashing a red light and go into denial. No, generally, we take the car to the mechanic or read the manual. The manufacturer should know best and so it is with God, our creator; He knows what is best. For so long, the Christian community has ignored the instructions our loving heavenly Father has given, and that is precisely why the body of Christ is more ill even than the world.

Let's Do a Review of What Has Been Uncovered

We have more people with flus, colds, and respiratory problems than ever before. One out of two Americans has cancer. One out of three has heart disease. Diabetes is on the rise and taking our nation to the brink. Depression, anxiety, and stress are major epidemics. Americans suffer primarily with low energy and chronic fatigue. What is this telling us and what do you think has caused this?

CHAPTER 3

Causes of the Chronic Epidemic of Degenerative Disease

Modern Medicine and Processed Food

Do you like watching the news on television? You can't watch television, though, without being inundated with all these toxic drug commercials that warn you if you take this, your liver may fall out, your bladder may explode, your heart may stop, your tongue may swell, but you will be *so* happy; at least you won't be depressed, but you might be suicidal! If you listen to these ads, you will soon realize that the bottom line is, "Stay drugged, America!" We have become a schizophrenic society—totally drugged. The spectrum isn't whether it is legal or illegal; we are a fully drugged society. This means we have become fully dependent on medications or drugs from one side or the other while believing we are health conscious. We are simply out of touch with ourselves. We have become mindless robots! Paul says, "Who has bewitched you?" (Galatians 3:1). How did this happen? How did we start on this path of destruction? It doesn't have to be this way; it can change if we wake up and become sober.

According to *Pill Poppers*, over the course of a lifetime, the average person may be prescribed fourteen thousand chemical pills, and this does not include over the counter medicine. By the time that most reach seventy, they are already on at least five synthetic chemicals (meds) daily. Is this God's plan for a long and healthy life? Are all of these meds beneficial since every single one has a toxic side effect, which sometimes is suicide or death? No drug is free of side effects. The side effects are then treated with more drugs so we have the vicious cycle to early disease and premature death. God has something better up His sleeve.

The world's current paradigm expects that you will get sick. This is not a good or healthy mindset. We expect to get colds and the flu. We expect, as we get older, to develop some chronic disease and die from it. And then, when we do get sick, unless we think we can help ourselves, we see the doctor. That's what I did when I became deathly ill from a poisoned health product from the health food store. But the medical community could offer me no hope. They did not have any medicine to cure my toxic, poisoned blood and muscles. Had I not had the knowledge of how the body can heal of just about any disease, I would have died along with the other 1,500 who did die. Most Americans do only what the doctors say to do medically. Remember, doctors are not trained in what heals the body. But many of us still accept what the doctor says and take the prescription. Most of the time, we are only treating the symptoms. The underlying problems are seldom addressed. Today's medicine expects us to get sick and then suppresses the symptoms of our illness.

Our bodies are self-repairing, self-energizing, and we weren't created to get sick. God created our bodies to heal themselves when we put in the correct ingredients. We were designed by God to live long lives *free of disease.*

There is much we need to unlearn that we have accepted as truth. So much of what we have heard is just myth. We don't have to expect to get colds and the flu or cancer. ***Disease should almost never happen.*** And that should be especially so if we know how to walk in health according to God's design.

How Has Our Diet in America Changed?

We are eating more and more fabricated and imitation foods. That means we are eating more and more of less and less. Fewer and fewer nutrients are reaching our cells with more and more calories. An ever-increasing proportion of the so-called food we eat is no longer even food. It is a high-priced chemistry experiment designed to simulate food. Some examples would be the non-dairy creamers, egg substitutes, margarines and spreads, artificial sweeteners, many breakfast cereals, and artificial fats that fall into this category. Some people think that frozen food is as good as fresh food. But, no it isn't; frozen food has been processed, and the nutrient content has been substantially reduced by the time you eat it.

As we have gone from a developing country to the present Westernized way of life, we have created the roots of our diet problems. From 1910 to 1976, we have increased our fat intake by 28 percent and decreased the carbohydrate intake by 45 percent and we have increased our sugar intake by 31 percent. As other countries around the world become more modernized, they progressively change to the Western diet. Consequently, where no degenerative disease existed, there now are diabetes and hypertension clinics.

The average diet for people in the United States now contains 3,100 calories, with 42 percent empty calories. Empty calories means there is no nutrient value in the food other than calories. Sugars and syrups account for 17 percent; fats and 18 percent oils; and alcoholic beverages 7 percent of the calories of the average diet. None of this contains any vitamins or minerals. In addition, about 17 percent of the diet is made of refined and partially refortified grains in the form of cereals and breads. About two-thirds of the sugar consumed in this country has been added to our processed food; the remainder is added to breakfasts, beverages, desserts, baked goods, and routine cooking. All together we are consuming over 150 pounds of sugar per person a year. I have more information on sugar and how it is impacting our health in the chapter called "Foods that Kill."

Sorcery, Witchcraft, and Pharmaceia

Prescription drugs cause about 350 deaths *daily*—not annually—but daily and cause about 13 percent of all birth defects. Do you really think they are the answer? Don't take these drugs unless you absolutely have to. It is best to seek alternative health professionals who can support you with a holistic nutritional plan.

In Mark 5:26, it mentions a woman who had suffered a great deal under the care of many doctors and had spent all she had, yet instead of getting better, she grew worse. And this is happening all the time today.

According to the New Testament, Paul strongly asks us, "Who has bewitched you?" Why would he ask this? Is it possible that believers can be very deceived?

God's heart is for us to thrive, not just survive. For that to happen, we must take responsibility for our own health and address the cause. When we run to the altar for prayer and do not address the cause, this can be witchcraft. When we run to our doctors and say, "I'm sick, please fix me, and please give me a pill," this too can be witchcraft. In Galatians 5 (the epistle of freedom in Christ), Paul warns us about pharmaceia, witchcraft, and sorcery. This doesn't mean we never pray or never take a pill, but neither gets to the cause. If we are going to walk in health for the long haul and fulfill our destinies, we will need to know the cause. What is causing my sickness that is within my control to change?

If the person you are praying for is blaming their disease on the devil, try asking them what they ate for breakfast that is creating a climate of disease in the body. With God's original health plan being the paradigm standard, do a little analysis on breakfast, lunch, and dinner. Now do you really think the devil is the culprit? Can we blame the devil for our sickness? Did the devil fix your breakfast? This will help them take responsibility for their own health. We can't grab something from the drive-through, eat sweet rolls, sausage, and bacon, and then blame our ill health on the devil. By the way, bacon is the most carcinogenic (cancer-causing) meat in the world. When we eat bacon, cold cuts, etc., we have a 6,700 percent greater chance of getting stomach and pancreatic cancer. The nitrates and nitrites create nitrosamines in the gut, which cause stomach, brain, and pancreatic cancer. And according to Ralph W. Moss, PhD, "Cancer risks lurk in hot dogs and burgers" (*Cancer Chronicles*, July 1994). It's been shown that children who eat twelve or more hot dogs a month have a 9.5 percent greater propensity of getting leukemia.

By the way, have you ever considered the connection between the FDA? It is aptly called the Food and Drug Administration for a reason.

Americans eat and drink popular foods that are laced with dangerous chemicals. Americans eat, on average, a staggering 193 pounds of food containing this chemical every year at levels thirteen times higher than those already linked to serious birth defects and a wide variety of chronic diseases. The chemical to which I am referring is glyphosate. This is the active ingredient in Monsanto's broad-spectrum herbicide Roundup. This chemical has estrogenic properties and drives breast cancer proliferation in the part per-trillion range. Back in February 2012, the journal *Archives of Toxicology* published a shocking study showing that Roundup is toxic to human DNA even when diluted to concentrations 450-fold lower than used in agriculture applications. It is always advisable to buy organic produce and even if you purchase the organic, still wash your produce with a surfactant cleaner, which removes all herbicides, pesticides, and chemicals. Even if you buy organic, you need to wash with our special surfactant cleaner because the workers urinate in the fields on that stuff! Yuk! This is a product we offer.

Have you ever noticed the commercials? Many times, the commercial is for a fast food restaurant, and then, the very next commercial is for a drug. The world assumes we will be sick and not take responsibility for living a healthy life. The commercial may be for a very spicy corn dog, for example, and then, the very next commercial is for Tums, Nexium, or Prilosec. And by the way, these medicines are not cheap; the pharmaceutical companies spend mere pennies to manufacture these, and they have an exorbitant markup.

This class of meds also blocks the assimilation of your nutrients

. . . because they are antacids.

What Has Caused All of This?

The world's medicine and the world's diet have become a way of life for believers. We are a set apart people for God's purposes. However, believers who would not think of getting drunk or committing adultery or murder have joined themselves with the diet of Egypt. They have stepped out from under God's protection, and it is deadly. It is cutting their destinies short when God has a work for each one of us. This way of eating has become a daily staple. We are living on the world's diet and the world's medicines. And consequently, we are suffering the world's diseases. Medicine is for the crisis; it is not intended to be a **daily staple.** Who would have ever thought about people living on artificial toxic substances called pharmaceuticals instead of eating what is right and good? If you are living on medicine, it is simply because you are not eating a diet that is healthy. It's that simple. When you step back from it, it is unbelievable, but like the frog in the pot, we have slowly accepted it, so we are dying when we don't have to.

We are eating the diet of Egypt, which is the standard American diet. We are also suffering the diseases of Egypt and being treated with the medicines of Egypt. We are then dying under the curse of three score and ten, which is the world's lifespan—the lifespan of Egypt. God told us He wants to deliver us from the diseases of Egypt; if we will listen, if we will obey, if we will do what He says, then *He will be our health*; thereby, we are delivered from the diseases of Egypt (Exodus 15:26). We easily quote that verse in the healing line *without the condition of "if."* Many are taking this verse out of context.

There is a lot of confusion with regard to this subject, so I want to refer to the Scripture for explanation.

In Galatians 3:1 it says, "Oh foolish Galatians, who has bewitched you? Who has cast an evil spell on you?"

Galatians 5:19-21 states, "Now the works of our flesh are manifest, which are these: adultery, fornication, uncleanness, lasciviousness, idolatry, witchcraft, hatred, strife, wrath, heresies, being envious or jealous, drunkenness, murder . . . " And then it continues to say, "they who do such things shall not see the Kingdom of God."

What is interesting is that Galatians is the book against legalism—the great book that establishes our freedom in Christ. But let me say that grace and mercy are not a license to sin. Paul says, "Shall we sin more that grace may abound? Absolutely not!" (Romans 6:1). God forbid. And so grace and mercy are not an excuse or license to sin.

Let's look at the word "witchcraft." This word is found only one time in the New Testament and that is in Galatians 5. In the Strong's Concordance, it is #5331. It is the word "Pharmaceia," and is taken from the root word #5332. The root word is *Pharmacuse*, which literally is translated into English as witchcraft; in the NIV, it is sorcery. In the New King James version, it is witchcraft and in the Amplified Bible, it is sorcery. The word for witchcraft in Galatians 5 is the same as medications prescribed by a pharmacist.

There is a place for medication and for medical doctors. But we should not be living on medical drugs as a way of life. Why? Because every medicine has a side effect, which will then precipitate taking another drug. Most people of all ages, who come to seek my counsel on their health, are already on a long list of medicines. This is not healthy and does not address the root cause of their condition. The Scripture says that every curse has a cause. It blocks the healing process, causing major toxic side effects for which the doctor will then prescribe more and more medications. They are deceptive; they keep the person from addressing the real cause and taking responsibility for what is making them sick. Medication is foreign to the human body. There is a place for medicine if we have been in an accident and are in pain, for example. There are cases where medicine may be needed to keep someone alive, but once they live, they do not need to be on medicine as a way of life.

The word witchcraft is the translation of the Greek word for Pharmaceia, which refers to the usage of drugs. It's from where our words pharmacy and pharmaceuticals come.

Also in Revelation 9:21 and 18:23, the word pharmaceia is associated with medicine, drugs, spells, poisoning, and witchcraft.

Medicine, processed junk foods, and fast food have replaced *real* food. They have become a daily staple and a household word. God gave us a grocery list for health and long life. If we want to live a long full healthy life, we must eat according to His design and provision. Live foods equal health and life; dead foods equal sickness and death. That's pure science. No one is putting a curse on us; we do that to ourselves by our own choices. Every curse has a cause; a curse causeless shall not alight (Proverbs 26:2). We are not talking about just an opinion but are addressing actual facts from medical journals.

Have you heard of three score and ten? Many believe that is how long we are to live. However, God says this is considered to be a curse. God intended man to live 120 years (Psalms 90:10 [Amplified] and Genesis 6:3). It's interesting that the average lifespan of Americans today is three score and ten (around seventy-eight) and by the time we reach three score and ten, research tells us Americans are on at least five pharmaceuticals. Despite all our medications and our healing lines, we do not feel well, and we are not well. Only about 5 percent of those prayed for get results. Why? While we are praying, our pantries and freezers are full of dead, devitalized foods and meats from animals that eat dead, diseased animals to clean up the planet. Our medicine chests are full of artificial substances foreign to our cells that promote death, not life. Every single medicine has a horrible side effect, and that even includes "baby aspirin," as innocent as that may sound. Many people, at the first sign of feeling bad, reach for the aspirin instead of asking what is making them sick. And so we suffer. Let's not have our heads in the sand; let's connect those dots!

I was watching the news the other night and a commercial came on for a particular medicine; then, they mentioned the side effects. It listed "death" as one of the possible side effects and said to call them if you experience any of these side effects. I believe the FDA thinks we are absolute idiots. The world assumes you will not want to take responsibility for your poor health, and they prey upon that. But are they right? *Next to salvation, there is no greater calling than to equip believers in walking in and sustaining their health.*

The doctor we have today is different from the one of our grandparents. Have we traded the personal, really connected doctor who was a friend that knew everything about us for a doctor who can only spend ten minutes with us and has all the latest high-tech pharmaceuticals at his fingertips? As one doctor told me, doctors have a pill for every ill, but every single one has at least one toxic side effect. How is this working for us? Is this a treat or a trick from the world's system?

Putting things in perspective, Dr. Gary Null says there is a gold standard with regard to medicine that is interesting, a golden rule within medicine. When a patient starts seeking some form of alternative treatment, let's say they have arthritis and they want to take fish oil or glucosamine, or let's say they have fibromyalgia (pains in their muscles) and they want to start taking cat's claw or turmeric. Let's say they have migraines and they want to take feverfew or B complex. They want to help themselves think well. They are tired of always being mentally fatigued and fogged so they start investigating lecithin or inositol for the health of the brain. The medical community says, "Stop, do not do that! First of all, there is no science behind it. Those who promote it are deceived. They are preventing you from proven therapies. If you have an enlarged prostate, do what the guy on television tells you to do . . . take the drug! If you have gastric reflux, take the purple pill! If you can't sleep at night, take that little thing where the fairy brings it into the window!" Medicine would say, "What we want you to do and remember is that we are science, we are the establishment, and we are MEDICINE. And for over 150 years, that has been the message and that's why at this point, *you only have about 5 percent of the American public actively leading healthy lives.*

Now, you have a lot of people exercising, you have a lot of people eating organic produce and you have probably over 60 percent of the adult American population taking some kind of a vitamin supplement each day. Then why is it that we rank 150th in the world in health? We are in the last 5 percent of happiness.

We Spend Two Trillion on Fighting Disease

Why is it that we spend 2 trillion dollars on fighting disease every year? To give you an idea, two trillion on disease is four times the entire defense budget. We spend more on disease than we do on food, defense, and housing combined each year. Why is it that a child has a better chance being born living a long and healthy life in Shanghai than in any city in the United States? Clearly, there is a difference between what we're being told versus what is being delivered.

It has been the official position of orthodox medicine that there is no association whatsoever between nutrition and one's health. In fact, the Arthritis Foundation and most doctors in general will say that there is nothing in the diet that will affect (either improve or cause) arthritic flare-ups or cancer or disease in general. And to check the proof of that mindset, Dr. Gary Null joined forces with Dr. Dorothy Smith of Cornell and Dr. Martin Seltman of Yale, both of whom have over sixty-five published papers in peer-reviewed journals and others of that same caliber. Their research focused on determining whether there is any documented, scientific benefit to vitamin supplementation. We have been told, "No, that's why the FDA is trying to regulate them." We are told by the medical establishment that if you take vitamins, you could have gotten the same thing from your foods, so why waste your money?

Dr. Gary Null and his team found 541,000 studies in peer-reviewed articles published by major institutions showing the science, efficacy, safety, and therapeutic dose range of a variety of vitamins. Who knew that there were over 26,000 studies on zinc and 28,000 studies on vitamin E and vitamin C? Clearly, the medical community didn't know this and the alternative community, with some exception, didn't either. No one knew that there was this enormous amount of positive information supporting these vitamins and minerals. This became one report proving that when people take their vitamins, their bodies reap tremendous benefit. But it had conveniently not been released.

Often I hear doctors say there is nothing you could have done to prevent your cancer. It's as if the cancer just flew in a window, and you caught it. Obviously, any doctor who makes a statement like that has not done his professional homework. I say, respectfully, he is ignorant. Over 1,400 studies show that those who eat a high fruit, vegetable, grain, bean, nut, and seed diet along with clean fish with fins and scales live longer lives. They called it the Mediterranean diet, and another name for it is the original Bible diet. *Interesting*.

Do You Want to Live Twenty-Nine Years Longer?

The studies proved that people eating this diet live twenty-nine years longer.

I don't know about you, but I love life, and I want to live. But it isn't just the diet. They found over two thousand studies in peer-reviewed journals that were about how we live, how we think, how good we feel, how much our belief systems empower us, how we deal with stress every day, how we are positive in the things we choose, and how we look for solutions and not just focus on the problems. All of these mean that we are living quality of life. The old idea that you can't be healthy until you're happy proved itself. Health and happiness are cousins, like the joy of the Lord is your strength. Vitamin L equals laughter.

An example is Norman Cousins, author of *Anatomy of an Illness*. He found that when orthodox medicine had nothing to help his debilitating conditions, laughter therapy did. I call that vitamin L. He would get old films of the Marx Brothers among others, and his laughter made him better. And then they found that laughter was connected to hormones. They found that every time you laugh and smile and every time you are in a beautiful environment or you are with someone you love, whether it's your brothers or sisters or children or spouse or dearly loved friends, it sets off positive hormones in the body. And these positive hormones give us this wonderful natural high (what is referred to as a "runners high"); the endorphins are pumping and we're feeling good. This just shows that we truly are what we think, believe, and accept. If you accept positive thoughts and reject negative ones, if you accept you can do things and reject that you can't, if you accept that you are a loving and beautiful person and not an ugly or negative person, if you accept that age is only a number, it doesn't matter how old you are. If you've lost none of your vitality, none of your emotional virility, none of your capacity to care about life and be creative, *then it doesn't matter what chronological age you are.*

Look at Picasso; look at the great painter, Grandma Moses. Look at all the people who did great work in the latter part of their lives. This is because they believed they could and were not dissuaded by the fact that they were old. They believed in themselves. Now there's a whole area of science showing that yes, it does matter what you think. Imagine the power of the mind. You do become what you believe. So now we know that when you believe positive things, when you put that energy into the universe, including prayer, it works!

Another reason for the sad status of health in our nation is that we have not been challenged to take charge of our health. We have abdicated that role mostly to doctors. This, again, is foolishness. Who has bewitched us? Did you know that medical doctors have not even been trained in health or nutrition? Would you call an electrician to fix your plumbing? But as long as we are living on meds, maybe we can't think straight, anyhow! Did you know that medical doctors are dying of the diseases we are trying to prevent because they are only preventable through good nutrition? Only one-fourth of our medical institutions offer one course in nutrition. The textbooks for medical schools are written and published by pharmaceutical companies. The pharmaceutical companies now own the television airways; that is why we are bombarded during the news with all kinds of brainwashing and lies about medicine.

CANCER: *Who is not living longer?*

CANCER: *Who is living longer?*

This was in the 1983 December issue of *Health Freedom News*. Dr. Hardin B. Jones, a prominent cancer researcher and former professor at the Donner Lab of Medical Physics at the University of California (at both Berkeley and Davis), stated that "People with cancer who submit to medical treatment live an average of three years. *People who develop cancer and refuse treatment live an average of 12.6 years longer.* Untreated patients live four times longer." Dr. Jones published these statistics in his article in *Transactions of the New York Academy of Science*, (Series 2, Vol. 18, No. 3, p. 322). This information can be found on numerous websites including www.brwwellness.com. This is not to say that there is not a place for medical treatment, but we need to know that these drugs can be lethal—even the label on the drug states that. We need to be knowledgeable about their limitations.

Remember: you are in charge of your health. Listen to your body and the wisdom within you. No one else is in charge of your body and your health, not even your doctor. He should be there to assist you in your getting well and healthy, but you are in charge. Again, Dr. Hardin Jones says, "My studies have proved conclusively that cancer patients who refuse chemotherapy and radiation actually live up to four times longer than treated patients."

The world assumes you will be sick. The world assumes you will be seduced by their dainties and not take personal responsibility for your own health. It assumes you will keep eating all the advertised foods and therefore need their pharmaceuticals. That is the best the world has to offer. Did you know there are nutrients that will heal you? God offers food and food supplements that heal you and give you a long and healthy quality of life with tons of fringe benefits and no toxic side effects.

The cure for cancer and all degenerative diseases is not found in a test tube, it is found in the kitchen, the cupboard, and the refrigerator! We have the cure. The cure for cancer and all other degenerative diseases is found in God's Word, and this is one of His top priorities (3 John 2). We need to take a fresh look at what the cures are for all these diseases. Hippocrates, the father of modern medicine, once said, "Your medicine will be your food, and your food will be your medicine." We cannot improve on that prescription. Thomas A. Edison once said, "The doctor of the future will give no drugs, but will interest his patients in the care of the human frame, diet, and in the cause and prevention of disease." Is your doctor doing that? Most medical doctors will say that there is no connection between what you eat and the disease you have.

The medical profession conditions us to treat the symptoms instead of questioning what is making us sick so we can deal with it!

Medicine and processed foods have become a way of life. We are a medicated society on legal drugs.

Let's consider what happens nutritionally in America on an average day. Then, we will consider an average day as to what Americans consume where medicine is concerned.

Let's Consider These Fast Food Facts

- 1,700,000 children eat at a hamburger chain.
- 27,000,000 eat at McDonald's daily.
- 10,000,000,000 Dunkin' donuts are served—that's 32 per person.
- 18,000,000,000 hot dogs are eaten (60 dogs per person a year).
- 100,000,000 M&Ms are sold.
- We drink 524,000,000 servings of Coke.
- 965,000 Americans drink Coke for breakfast.
- Americans spend $10,411,000 on potato chips.
- We spend $5,800,000 on cat food.
- We spend $8,550,000 on dog food.
- We spend $434,000,000 on toys.
- Americans only spend 3,700,000 on vitamins.
- We spend $2 billion on Easter candy annually.

Incidentally, pediatricians say this is the busiest time of the year for them—Easter and Halloween.

A quick look at these numbers will immediately tell you that Americans eat an unhealthy diet. There is a problem when we spend more on cat and dog food than we do on vitamins and healthy foods that promote optimal health and prevent disease. In fact, we spend three times more on potato chips and 117 times more on toys! Sometimes, it is a matter of priority. Is it any wonder that 28 percent of men and 34 percent of women are obese? It is estimated that obesity has cost the nation $117 billion in one year. This amount is rapidly closing in on the $140 billion in costs associated with smoking.

Often, I have heard people say that eating healthily is just too expensive. When I hear comments like that, I want to say, "Have you priced prostate cancer lately?" It costs at least $30,000 if the cancer has metastasized. I can't reiterate enough the current statistic that the average cancer patient spends $50,000 in his lifetime on cancer treatment and poor quality of health. Organic zinc and saw palmetto are two nutrients that are needed for the prostate. How expensive are they? They cost pennies, and think of the quality of health when you protect that important organ. I have a friend whose husband has cancer. She went to pick up one of the medications prescribed for him and it cost $1,000 to fill it, and that was "out of pocket"! There is one aspect of the cancer treatment story that is an unqualified success, and that is cancer's billion dollar profit margin. Keep in mind that chemo drugs can cost $10,000, $20,000, and even $30,000 a month. The average cancer patient will spend $50,000 on cancer in his or her lifetime. The treatment costs for just the top cancers have topped $56 billion annually, and total cancer care now exceeds $110 billion per year. Cancer is a big business. Are you one who says, "Oh well, my insurance will pay for that"? And that is exactly one of the reasons the drug and pharmaceutical cartels are taking this nation to the brink. There is a better way. It is called taking responsibility for our own health and taking the neutraceuticals that we need for optimal health and strength. The body is created to run on these according to God's design.

Where's the beef?

The Golden Arches are telling us where!

The cross has always been the world's symbol. However, someone reminded me that the cross has been replaced with the golden arches, which are now all over the world.

Americans eat nearly 50 billion hamburgers a year.

On average, we eat three hamburgers per week.

So that's 156 burgers per person per year.

On average, Americans eat three times more meat than people in other countries.

From the end of World War II to the mid 1970s, beef consumption per person doubled.

The US is now the largest beef producer in the world.

Our beef industry is a $74 billion per year powerhouse. It provides millions of jobs.

A Quarter Pounder at a fast food restaurant costs about $3 or $4 per burger. That's pretty cheap. But what we don't pay for at the counter, we end up paying for in other ways. There are many hidden costs. God intended man to live on fresh fruits, vegetables, whole grains, and raw nuts and seeds. The cow was allowed for the celebrations, maybe once a year or once every five years. Instead, Americans are eating a lot more than what was intended and what is actually healthy.

People often tell me they don't know why they had a stroke or have cancer or why they don't feel well. Then they say, "But I eat really well!" To which I ask, "What did you have for dinner last night?" It's usually revelatory to them that they are not eating as healthily as they had thought.

Consider, for example, the BK Quad Stacker. Here's what you get on one sandwich: four hamburger patties, four slices of cheese, eight strips of bacon, sauce, and a bun for almost a thousand calories. The BK Quad Stacker contains 1.5 days of saturated fats . . . thirty grams of saturated fat and three grams of the highly dangerous fats. It also has more than a day's sodium intake for anyone over fifty (1,800 milligrams).

We have the best medical technology in the world—this country is the place to be if you need a hospital. If you have an eye socked out, need a bone set, need to have a baby, have some tests run, this is the best nation medically to be. Twenty percent of medicine is good. *But 80 percent is failing miserably.* When doctors begin to give advice on health, they often fail to provide accurate advice. *Doctors are not trained in health.* Doctors are trained in managing your sickness with medical drugs and surgery. Neither of which is the total answer for health and longevity. Many medical doctors are dying of the same diseases we are teaching people to prevent.

Americans have turned over the care of their health to their medical doctors and the pharmaceutical industry. These industries are taking our nation to the brink.

In all fairness, doctors are not trained in health. Their textbooks are written by pharmaceutical companies. Only one-fourth of our medical institutions have one course in nutrition. Doctors are trained to manage your sickness. One med leads to another because of the terrible side effects of every drug. I see young people already on a long list of the world's meds.

If medicine were the answer, we'd be the healthiest nation in the world. Instead, we are one of the sickest. Let's consider a daily medical profile: To cure our ills, we take billions of drugs every year. Over a million people a year end up in the hospital as a result of negative reactions to drugs. We are a medicated society because of legal unsafe drugs.

Let's Sum Up a Daily Medical Profile

To cure our ills, we have entrusted our health to our medical doctor. We take trillions of dollars of drugs every year. Over a million people a year end up in the hospital as a result of negative reactions to drugs. Don't forget that Vioxx (that's just one drug) killed forty-three thousand people and the pharmaceutical company knew that it was unsafe. Is there a better way? And do you really want to put your life in the hands of people like this? Do you think their motive in life is to improve your health?

Consider the following daily statistics:
- One of the main reasons why Americans see a doctor is low energy.
- Another main reason why Americans see a doctor is for neuropathy (pain).
- 220,000 Americans see a doctor just because of headaches.
- 80,000,000 tablets of aspirin are consumed.
- $1,400,000 is spent on laxatives.
- $2.6 billion goes to over the counter pain relievers.
- $45.2 million is spent on prescription drugs.
- 2 million Americans suffer heartburn.
- $290 million is paid to doctors.
- 4,000 Americans have a heart attack.
- 1,500 Americans die from a heart attack.
- Our prostates are costing $16,000 for treatment if the cancer has not metastasized. If it is cancer and has metastasized, the treatment of surgery is $30,000.

(By the time you are reading this, statistics could have changed; nevertheless, they are offered to give a perspective on the choices we are making with regard to taking charge of our health. Unfortunately, the

statistics are worsening with time.)

Sometimes we need drugs for the crisis, but they are not intended for the long haul, especially since every drug is a poison and has a toxic side effect. They are not natural to the body, and to be dependent on them as a daily staple is not the best way to live. Drugs can keep us alive sometimes, but they do not promote quality of health and long life. Do you really want to live to one hundred hooked up to machines or even in a wheelchair if you can help it? If you start early enough, you can help it. In fact, if you are still breathing, it is not too late to start.

And I hear people say that vitamins are expensive! Americans spend more on almost everything other than health and good vitamins. They spend more on chips, candy, toys, their cars, vacations, and cat food than they do on good vitamins. I think it can be *simply a matter of priority.* Remember, nothing can be fully enjoyed apart from your health. Do you really think this is the answer to health or is there a better way? Do you think it would be a good idea to budget in some resources toward your health?

According to the FDA, there were 14 million prescriptions written in the U.S. for antidepressants in 1992. In 2002, just ten years later, that number had jumped to 157 million prescriptions. Eleven million of those were prescribed for children under the age of eighteen, some as young as two to four years old.

Consider what happened with one drug. Vioxx caused the deaths of 43,000 Americans. On November 18, 2004, Dr. David Graham, a twenty-year veteran Food and Drug Administration (FDA) scientist, rocked the pharmaceutical industry with Senate testimony that shook six multinational corporations. It drew vital public attention to the secret life inside the FDA, and stopped the sales of a deadly, but hugely popular, arthritis medication. His testimony exposed tragic public health consequences stemming from a legalized conflict of interest; the FDA is one of the few government agencies whose funding depends largely on the success of products of the industry it regulates. Due to Graham's appearance, the deadly market for pain relievers will never be the same.

Let's Look at the Markup on Some Very Popular Drugs:

Celebrex 100 mg (possible side effects are swelling of the lips, fingers, chest pain)
Consumer pays $130.27 (100 tablets)
Pharmaceutical company pays $0.60 to make
Markup is 21,712 percent

Claritin 10 mg (possible side effects are headaches, pharyngitis, diarrhea)
Consumer pays $217.17 (100 tablets)
Pharmaceutical company pays $0.71 to make
Markup is 30,306 percent

Norvasec 10 mg (possible side effects are difficulty breathing, redness of the face, swelling of the feet)
Consumer pays $188.29 (100 tablets)
Pharmaceutical company pays $0.14 to make
Markup is 134,493 percent (talk about a markup!) This is criminal!

Prevacid 30 mg (possible side effects are anxiety, nausea, diarrhea)
Consumer pays $44.77 (100 tablets)
Pharmaceutical company pays $1.01
Markup is 34,136 percent

Prilosec 20 mg (side effects are osteoporosis and diarrhea)
Consumer pays $360.97 (100 tablets)
Pharmaceutical company pays $0.52
Markup is 69,417 percent

Prozac 20 mg (side effects are irregular heartbeat, anxiety, lack of concentration)
Consumer pays $247.47 (100 tablets)
Pharmaceutical company pays $0.11

Markup Is 224,973 percent

Xanax 1 mg (side effects are loss of memory, sad, changes in speech)
Consumer pays $136.79 (100 tablets)
Pharmaceutical company pays $0.02
Markup is 569,958 percent

Zoloft 50 mg (possible side effects include suicide and tremors)
Now, that can be depressing!
Consumer pays $206.87
Pharmaceutical company pays $1.75
Markup is 11,821 percent

Zocor 40 mg (possible side effect of this statin drug is breakdown of muscle tissue leading to kidney failure)
Your cholesterol may improve but you lose your kidneys . . . what a deal!!!!!
Consumer pays $350.27 (100 tablets)
Pharmaceutical company pays $8.63
Markup is 4,059 percent

Vasotec 10 mg (possible side effect is blurred vision, confusion, lightheadedness, and unusual fatigue, just to name a few)
Consumer pays $102.37 (100 tablets)
Pharmaceutical company pays $0.20
Markup is 51,185 percent

Does this disturb you as it does me? I think this is criminal. Where is the outcry?

So what we have is an extreme profit—more than any other industry, more than any other industry of which I am aware. And this has been done by people who have committed massive crimes against humanity and gotten a clean bill of health for it. These people continually tell us that their vaccines are safe and effective. But they have no double-blind, placebo-controlled studies (these are studies that are to be used to guard against bias and placebo effects) and they are willing to allow the most vulnerable among us—children, pregnant women, and seniors—to get this vaccine. I am not opposed to any vaccine that can be shown to be safe and effective. I am opposed to science that is so faulty, so ridden with inconsistencies and contradictions, that it does not align with the truth. The industry is not open to allowing people to make their own choices. This information is not a secret but is in view of all of the public.

Freedom Of Choice

I heard someone say, "I am a healthy American, and as such, I do not want to put a toxic drug in my body." I concur that is a violation of my constitutional right, as well as decency and ethics.

All of these medicines are extremely expensive on a monthly basis. Since 1998, drug companies have spent $758 million on lobbying—more than any other industry, according to government records analyzed by the Center for Public Integrity, a watchdog group. In Washington, the industry has 1,274 lobbyists—more than two for every member of Congress. That is over half a billion dollars that have a dramatic influence on how drugs are viewed politically. When Senator Bill Frist needed help in November for a quick tour celebrating the victories of newly elected Republican senators, he didn't have to look far. A Gulfstream corporate jet owned by drug maker Schering-Plough was ready to zip the senate majority leader to stops in Florida, Georgia, and the Carolinas. Frist's political committee reimbursed the drug maker $10,809, the equivalent of a first-class fare for the same trip on a commercial airline, as campaign rules require. The price, a fraction of the cost of a charter flight, was almost a wash for Frist; Schering had donated $10,000 to his committee in 2003-2004. What he got was worth far more: the convenience, luxury, and efficiency of flying on his own schedule.

The drug company's friendly gesture toward the Senate's most powerful member at the time illustrates the political clout of the pharmaceutical industry. It will be needed in the months ahead as the industry faces the threat of increased federal regulation, brought on by mounting concerns about the safety of the nation's drug supply. The drug company's corporate planes have been made available to not only Frist but also to dozens of other powerful lawmakers. Former House Speaker Dennis Hastert, R-Ill., took at least four trips to GOP fund-raising events in two years aboard Pfizer's Gulfstream.

Drug companies and their officials contributed at least $17 million to federal candidates in some of the elections, including nearly $1 million to President Bush and more than $500,000 to his opponent, John Kerry. At least eighteen members of Congress received more than $100,000 apiece.

Over 225,000 people die each year from medical and physician error or adverse reactions to drugs or surgery.

An interesting consideration is that as we look around the world, we see societies where medicine is very prominent, and these are some of the sickest nations in the world.

Conversely, the nations that are rather ignorant about how to care for the body, medically speaking, are some of the healthiest nations in the world.

And to prove this point, there have been four medical doctor strikes in recent years. Two, here in the US; one in Israel; one in Canada; and another one in South America. In these cities where the medical strikes took place, that means the doctors did not show up either at their hospitals or their offices, and the death rate dropped substantially between 40 and 60 percent! In 1976, the mortality rate in Bogotá, Columbia, dropped 37 percent during a fifty-two day strike by doctors. In Los Angeles, California, the death rate dropped 18 percent during a doctor's strike in 1976. The most amazing of all was a strike in 1973 in Israel, where the mortality rate dropped 50 percent during a two-month strike. Morticians complained that "business hadn't been this slow since the last doctor's strike twenty years ago." All of this was because the doctors were not there prescribing drugs and cutting people open. Yet, despite these facts, most Americans still place their health in the hands of individuals who have proven themselves unworthy of this trust. Most doctors are using harmful drugs with side effects. This is the reason they are labeled prescription drugs and not sold over the counter. Rarely do they counsel their patients on the dangers of white sugar, artificial sweeteners, white flour, white table salt, or preservatives in food. Nor is anything said about eating sausage, ham, bacon, pepperoni, and shellfish, a few of the foods that are killing us.

When the doctors went on strike, people could not get their harmful drugs, so they had to take the responsibility of health into their own hands.

I am not saying we are not thankful for doctors or that we should do away with them. But I do believe we need to re-evaluate how doctors are practicing and realize they are not God. We must not be in denial about their limitations. As a believer, I cannot afford to have my head in the sand or be so heavily drugged on **legal drugs** that I don't have the mind of Christ and can't think straight. The Scriptures warn us to be sober and alert because we have an enemy that comes to rob, kill, and destroy (John 10:10).

It has been said that on one of the pyramids, it states, "One-fourth of what we eat feeds our bodies, and three-fourths goes to feed our doctors."

Who is responsible for your health? Your spouse? Your best friend? Your pastor? What about your doctor?

Many Americans are happy to take their symptoms to their doctor, plop them on his lap, and say, "Fix me. I'll pay you anything, Doctor, if you will give me my health back." But your doctor cannot do it. Health is not found in a medicine, pharmaceutical drug, or a test tube. But instead, health is found in God's prescriptions: "Come, buy food and wine without price; ones that are good for you" (Isaiah 55:2). Most doctors know nothing about neutraceuticals that are both natural to the human body and good and healthy for you.

I am all for doctors exercising their gifts where they are trained, but doctors have stepped over the line in telling people what to do about cancer, heart disease, diabetes, arthritis, osteoporosis, etc. These diseases are coming from what we put in our bodies, and that is what must be addressed to prevent or heal those top killers. They are not trained in the healing or prevention of disease. Once they give a diagnosis, it needs to stop right there. Instead, they prescribe very strong, toxic medicines as a way of life, not just for the crisis. Doctors are dying of these diseases themselves.

CHAPTER 4

Cultures That Are
Living Longer

If we rank 150th in world health, what are some of the cultures that are among the healthiest, and *what do they eat in contrast to what we eat?* Could it be that their lifestyles are lining up with God's original health plan? And yet most would not claim to be a Christian nation.

I am not telling you that to be healthy you must be a vegetarian. But I will say that vegetarians are among some of the healthiest and longest living people on Earth. Isn't it interesting that the original health plan is fresh fruits, vegetables, whole grains, raw nuts, and raw seeds?

When God introduced a little bit of clean meat into our diet, do you know what transpired?

Obviously, God did not confer with the Dairy Council or the Cattlemen's Association when He introduced His nutritional plan. But it is really curious that after the flood, God introduced a *little bit* of clean animal protein. And do you know what happened? The ages of the patriarchs began to decline at that time from 900 to 700 and on down until now, where it is 120. It sounds like eating meat can be dangerous! I am not necessarily saying not to eat meat, but most of us know that Americans eat too much meat three meals a day, and it is often the wrong kind—the animals God said would make you sick if you eat them and that was *for all the generations to come*—I believe that includes us.

When God introduced a little bit of meat, He really intended it to be for the celebrations, not as a daily staple. "Kill the fatted calf for the celebration or feast." You will note it does not say kill the fatted PIG, HOG, or SWINE. Those are the animals He sends demons into! What does that tell you about what Jesus thinks about the pig? He certainly did not and does not endorse eating a pig. But most believers do. Now Americans call the pig delicious pepperoni, honey baked ham, bacon, sausage, pork chops, etc. Christians eat the most unholy meat on the most holy day of the year! In another chapter we will discuss that food group we call meat and dairy for clarification of which meat we can eat a little bit of and which to never eat unless we want to be sick.

What about Some of the Other Cultures?

Let me acquaint you with a great example. In his tapes "Never Be Sick Again," Raymond Francis shares about a medical researcher who interviewed a 133-year-old farmer in Vilcabamba who still works his farm every day. He is a healthy, functional certifiably 133-year-old man. At the time of the interview, he was still working his farms on the steep slopes of a mountain on a daily basis. He had fathered his last child at age 107. He had every tooth in his mouth (the health of our teeth and gums is a telltale sign of how healthy we really are). He was cognitively sharp. The research doctor asked if he had ever been sick. And the man answered, "Oh yes, I have been sick; I've had several colds." Let's note that this was several colds in 133 years. His idea of being sick was having a cold. These people die of old age well beyond one hundred. They do not die of chronic degenerative diseases. In other words, **they don't get sick in order to die.** Most Americans experience several colds every year. According to the CDC, there are as many as a billion colds in the US, and 4,500 people die annually from influenza due to the common cold. Now, that's nothing to sneeze at! So it is all about how we build our immune systems.

When we examine the diet of developing countries of the world where degenerative disease is rare, we find they rely on complex carbohydrates with very little refined food, a very little bit of meat, if any, and a low calorie diet of two thousand calories or less a day along with an active life. Conversely, our diet is very refined, fatty, and consists of about three thousand daily calories with a very sedentary lifestyle.

Some examples of these other cultures would be the Russian Caucasians, the Yucatan Indians, the East Indian Todas, and the Pakistan Hunzakuts—who live to be ninety to one hundred years old. Vilcabamba is home to one of the cultures that live the longest. Vilcabamba is a small village in southern Ecuador located in an elevated valley. The valley is extremely inaccessible and has therefore been protected from many modern influences such as prepackaged foods and preservatives. Vilcabambas claim an extremely long life, and most importantly, good health throughout their entire existence. And that is our inheritance. The people of Vilcabamba have been in the eye of many scientists since the mid 1950s. Members of their community have appeared in *Ripley's Believe it or Not* and been featured in *National Geographic, Reader's Digest,* and other popular press outlets. The researchers have documented very little chronic illness, even for the oldest of the Vilcabamba people.

How do they stay healthy? What is their secret? An international conference in 1978 concluded that the Vilcabambas remain healthy because they are lean, eat a healthy diet, have low cholesterol, and are very active throughout their long lives.

So What Do They Eat?

Vegetables picked fresh from the garden, eaten the same day. They also eat fruits right off the trees. Whole grains, seeds, and nuts are also part of the Vilcabamba diet. There are almost no animal products to be found in their diet and no packaged or prepared food. Sounds just like the Bible diet to me! That's God's grocery list for health (Genesis 1:29 and 30).

Do They Exercise?

Their daily lives are filled with hiking up the slopes to harvest foods, cleaning, cultivating vegetables, and picking fruits. There is no such thing as formal exercise, but rather a life full of activity.

How Are the Elderly Treated in Vilcabamba?

They are treated wonderfully. Just that fact alone makes me want to move there. The way they are treated by their children and grand-children contributes to their overwhelmingly positive health. Aging is seen as a grace, and people are given more respect as they grow older. It is said that the Vilcabamba actually look forward to getting old, to becoming more mature, and to growing as a person. They have a lot of laughter and joy in their lives. Let's connect some dots here. Doesn't God's Word say the joy of the Lord is your strength?

What about the Hunzas?

This is an area in the northern tip of Pakistan. The Hunzas are con-sidered to be some of the healthiest people on Earth. It is believed that among these people, centenarians are a common occurrence, and that it is not unusual for an elderly person to reach the venerable age of 130. It has even been reported that a significant number have sur-vived to the incredible age of 145! They exist isolated from the rest of the world in the Himalayan Mountains where they live to be 100 to 120 years of age. They have no cancer, heart attacks, or other major disorders. They are active and fit to the end of their lives. Overweight people are unheard of because they have the perfect weight control system.

The Hunzas eat fruits and vegetables. They eat barley, millet, buck-wheat, and wheat. The Hunzas are not completely vegetarian, but meat forms a minimal part of their daily diet. Their main staples are raw yogurt; whole grains, such as barley, wheat, buckwheat; fruits, mostly apricots, apples, and grapes; and assorted vegetables eaten mostly raw. They consume a little bit of raw goat's milk. They eat fertile eggs and very little animal protein and only the clean meat (no pork and no shellfish) for the celebrations, perhaps only once a month. They eat the original health plan Bible diet, also known as the Mediterranean diet.

Many laboratory tests have been conducted to compare the strength and stamina of meat eaters against vegetarians. Yale professor Irving Fisher selected men from three groups: meat-eating athletes, vegetarian athletes, and vegetarian sedentary subjects. He found that the meat-eating athletes showed far less endurance than even the sedentary vegetarians. Dr. J. Ioteyko of Paris performed a comparable study and found that vegetarians averaged two to three times more stamina than meat eaters. He also found that vegetarians only took one-fifth of the time to recover from exhaustion than did their meat-eating counterparts.

A Danish study in 1968 revealed that men peddling on a stationary bicycle until muscle failure lasted an average of 114 minutes on a mixed meat and vegetable diet, 57 minutes on a high meat diet, and a whopping 167 minutes on a strict vegetarian diet according to John Robbins, *Diet for New America* (p. 156-158).

Israel, of course, is a wonderful example of health and longevity. Israel does not claim to be a Christian nation. They don't have healing lines, but they do take Jehovah God seriously when it comes to what they eat. Healing lines are wonderful if you need them, but Israel typically doesn't need them when it comes to their health.

Other cultures that are noteworthy are the Maya Indians of Yucatan. They are of Semitic origin. Their diet is low in animal protein and high in complex carbohydrates. The Maya are primarily vegetarian.

Bulgarians are among the healthiest in Europe, and they possess great vitality and longevity. Bulgaria has more people over one hundred years old than any other country in the world. What do they eat? They eat very little meat; they eat black bread and vegetables. I refer to this passage that actually mentions those very healthy foods (2 Samuel 17:28) which are wheat, barley, meal, parched grain, beans, lentils, peas, honey, curds, and sheep.

Our bodies were created to live to be 120 to 150 (Genesis 6:3). Often I hear people ask about the three score and ten in Psalm 90. They assume that is the lifespan we are given biblically. However, look at the footnote in that context which says that this is considered to be a curse; God intended man to live 120 years.

The lifespan in America is around seventy-two to seventy-eight, and that correlates with the three score and ten curse. Dying in our seventies correlates to the standard American diet and lifestyle, which shortens our lifespan and destinies. Three score and ten is the world's lifespan, which is the curse. God intended man to live to 120.

CHAPTER 5

Foods That Heal (Eat As If Your Life Depends on It)

God's Grocery List
What's in God's Grocery Cart?
God's Groceries are a Mighty Weapon Against Sickness and Disease

Eat as if your life depends on it, because it does! So many are eating as if it doesn't matter what we put in our bodies. Are we just accepting disease as a way of life?

It's time for the body of Christ to start taking degenerative diseases more seriously throughout our lives and not just once it's too late. Even starting in our 30s, 40s, and 50s, the choices we make with our daily food can *PREVENT* these terrible diseases.

Eating properly as if your life depends on it is a mighty weapon given to us by God against sickness and disease. You say, "But I don't like vegetables." And I say, "You might have to learn to like cobalt," which is one of the treatments, among others, for cancer. The power of life and death is in the tongue—not only in what we say but also in what we are putting in our mouths and eating and drinking.

Every one of us has to deal daily with food, just like we have to deal wisely with finances. God wants more than anything else for us to prosper in our health and in our finances (3 John 1:2). They are both extremely important while we are on the earth. And it is important that we learn the truth about both and deal wisely with both. We can choose blessings instead of curses.

God's Word says if you eat certain foods, you will be sick. Leviticus 11 gives us a list of animals that if eaten will be an abomination (disease) to you. It's interesting that these animals are the very ones that Americans are eating sometimes even three times a day. In that kind of a diet, where would we be getting the antioxidants to prevent cancer and premature aging, the fiber to cleanse the body of toxins, and the enzymes to prevent cancer? None of these can be found in animal meat and dairy.

Life is a choice. Health is a choice. Health is not by accident. We don't just accidentally fall into health. No, it is by intentionality. God created our bodies to be in health.

I encourage you to choose health and long life.

God gave us the original health plan that is just as healthy and applicable today as it was four thousand years ago. Studies show that it can easily add twenty-nine years and more to your life; that's good news! God is the same yesterday, today, and forever, and He has not changed in His instructions for His children for all the generations to come. The cultures that follow His guidelines for health for the most part are not Christian nations or cultures, yet they do not have heart disease, cancer, diabetes, etc., and they are living to one hundred and beyond.

If eating a diet of fresh fruits and vegetables is what we should be doing, let's have a look at what we actually are doing. According to the U.S. Bureau of Labor Statistics, the average US household now spends $4,399 per year on food. Out of more than $4,000 spent on food, only $132 a year is spent on fresh fruits and vegetables. We don't need to look any further as to why we are so sick in our nation and in the body of Christ.

Foods That Heal

These are the food groups that are rich in phytonutrients. These are foods that are right in our supermarkets. If you switch to organically grown foods, this will cut your toxic intake. The rule of thumb is to shop around the perimeter of the store where the fresh fruits and vegetables are displayed. Then promptly leave unless you need some staples or cleaning products from the center aisles of the store.

Acid and alkaline:
PHydrion strips:
5.5 is the range
7.4 is normal
Urine has a wider range of 4.5-8

There are foods we eat that are acid and those that are alkaline. What is the difference? The standard American diet is very acidic, which creates a bio-terrain of disease. The healthiest eating plan is alkaline. God's original health plan for His children for ALL THE GENERATIONS TO COME is alkaline. That would be fresh fruits, vegetables, whole grains, raw nuts, and raw seeds. But not Planters Roasted Mixed Nuts or peanuts! When we roast a nut, it becomes rancid, or a hydrogenated oil, which can cause colon cancer, prostate cancer, and breast cancer.

Please note an interesting study from the *Archives of Internal Medicine*. This is a study of almost four hundred thousand men and women between the ages of fifty to seventy-one talking about the importance of eating the Mediterranean diet. Studies show that eating the Mediterranean diet adds twenty-nine years to your lifespan.

If you follow the guideline of five is fine and nine is divine, the number of servings of fresh fruits and vegetables you should be consuming daily, you come pretty close to the Mediterranean diet. Sometimes even just little changes can make a huge difference. If that is difficult for you, we carry a capsule which contains the seed benefit of thousands of carrots, cherries, and more (Genesis 1:29, 30).

The Mediterranean diet is rich in fish with fins and scales (with no hormones or antibiotics), fruit and vegetables, raw nuts, raw seeds, and whole grains. However, it is low in dairy and meat.

What has been discovered from this study is that you are 21 percent less likely to die over a five-year period if you are consuming the Mediterranean diet. This diet is rich in antioxidants, for example (vitamins A, C, and E), which protect you from disease. Proper supplementation and wholesome nutrition can help you control your medical problems to where you may not even require medications.

Antioxidants Keep Us from Rusting Out!

Antioxidants are so important. Nature gave us antioxidants as a natural way to protect our cells. But they are not in meat and they are not in dairy and they are not in cookies and they are not in breads, crackers, chips, and all the things that Americans tend to predominantly eat. Instead, they are in the food groups of which we eat the least. They are raw vegetables and raw fruits. Selectively supplementing with this can help enormously. Organic produce is key.

The National Cancer Institute has said, "Diets rich in fruits and vegetables reduce the risk of cancer and other degenerative diseases." Why? Because they are rich in antioxidants.

In my nutritional practice, I offer a daily pack of vitamins, which contains twenty-six antioxidants in each daily pack. This is an easy way to get in a dosage of antioxidants that you can't get in your food alone today.

Research indicates that the less animal protein and dairy you consume, the healthier you are. And interestingly, the more plant foods you consume, the healthier you are as well.

The Cure for Cancer

Cancer cannot exist where there is oxygen in the bloodstream and in the cells.

God's groceries are chock full of antioxidants

Why is that? Because these foods are packed with antioxidants, which give you oxygen, and *cancer cannot exist where there is oxygen in the cells.* Do you see people running for a cure for cancer? God gave us the cure for cancer four thousand years ago. And to prove that point, *Dr. Warburg won his first Nobel Prize in 1931 for proving cancer is caused by a lack of oxygen respiration in cells. He stated in an article titled "The Prime Cause and Prevention of Cancer" that "the cause of cancer is no longer a mystery; we know it occurs whenever any cell is denied 60 percent of its oxygen requirements."*

God's Groceries are Chock-Full of the Right Kind of Fiber

The foods listed below are packed with fiber. The Cancer Institute says we need twenty-five to thirty grams of fiber daily to prevent one of our top killers (colon cancer), but God told us to eat this way four thousand years ago. Medical science is always having to catch up with God's Word. The original health plan is rich in live enzymes. Cancer, without being overly simplified, is a pancreatic enzyme deficiency.

Other compounds called phytochemicals that help protect your DNA and fight free-radical damage are found only in plant foods. They are not in meat or dairy.

What are some of these powerhouse foods that studies have demonstrated play an important role in our health?

God's Original Health Plan Is Found in Genesis 1:29, 30

These foods are your key to total health. Of course, because our country has not been obedient to God's principles of health, we must supplement today with selective organic supplements in addition to improving our diets.

What does God's grocery list of foods do for you? These are the raw and living foods:
- They cleanse and detoxify the system
- Replenish the cells
- Revitalize the cells of the body
- These are living foods that are eaten in their raw state
- They are not cooked over 118 degrees
- These foods contain oxygen, and cancer cannot exist where there is oxygen in the cells

These are the foods that can prevent and heal the following:
- Cancer
- Eye Problems
- Fatigue
- Fibrocystic Breast Disease
- Uterine Fibroids
- Endometriosis
- Varicose Veins
- PMS
- Hot Flashes
- Macular Degeneration
- Heart Disease
- Memory And Brain Issues (Foggy Thinking)
- Diabetes
- Arthritis
- Hearing Loss
- Hair Loss
- Liver Health
- Thyroid Health

Would you like to prevent or heal any of those diseases?

I heard an MD say, "I have never pulled a stalk of broccoli out of a clogged artery." Then he proceeded to tell what he did pull out of a clogged artery, for example, long yellow strings or worms of hardened mucous. This is what you call arteriosclerosis!

Meat and dairy contribute to clogged arteries and hardening of the arteries. And this is the exact cause of heart conditions, cancer, strokes, and yes, even "senior moments." When the arteries to the brain are clogged, it blocks the flow of oxygen, which affects our memory and recall.

Let's note some of the foods on God's grocery list; consider why they are healthy and how many servings daily we should eat.

It is noteworthy that God's eating plan is not just a suggestion, but rather, a command. It is also noteworthy that when He gave His permission to eat meat, it was just that. He only gave His permission to eat a little bit of clean animal protein. But what do Americans eat a lot of? They eat a lot of meat, generally three meals a day, and many times, it is the meat that He said would kill us. When He gave us permission to eat a little bit of clean animal meat, the ages of the patriarchs began to decline from 900 to 700 and on down until now the lifespan for man is 120 years. Maybe we need to think twice before we eat three meals a day of meat.

God's original health plan does not cost trillions of dollars a year. We need to go back to the basics . . . and the beginning.

And God said, "Behold, I have given you every herb-bearing seed which is upon the face of the earth, and every tree, in the which is the fruit of a tree yielding seed; to you it shall be for food" (Genesis 1:29).

Some examples would be:

Whole grains: 6-11 servings daily (one serving is ½ cup)

- Wheat (not Wheat Thins) Note that much of the wheat today in our nation is genetically modified.
- Corn (not corn chips) However, the corn in our nation is GMO and not healthy now.
- Rye
- Barley
- Rice (not white rice)
- Millet
- Oats (not instant—preferably steel-cut oats)
- Buckwheat

Arrowhead Mills is a good brand you can trust.

Nature gives us another rich class of greens known as "super foods." These include long grasses like barley and rye, and rich green herbs like alfalfa. These foods are overflowing with healthy phytonutrients, amino acids, enzymes, antioxidants, vitamins, minerals, and phytochemicals.

Raw seeds:

- Sunflower
- Sesame

- Flax
- Pumpkin

Legumes:
- Soybeans (non GMO)
- Lentils
- Peas
- Other beans

Succulent foods (containing seeds):
- Eggplant
- Okra
- Bell pepper
- Squash
- Green beans
- Pumpkins
- Cucumbers
- Tomatoes
- Melons

And every tree in which the fruit of a tree yields seed. This category is the woody, perennial plants, shrubs, or bushes.

Some examples are:

Fruit trees: 2–4 servings daily (one serving is ½ cup)
- Citrus fruits
- Sub-acid fruits
- Sweet fruits
- Neutral fruits

A little tip here: I am sure you have peeled off those little stickers that are on every piece of fruit and vegetable in the market. Do you know what those numbers mean? You can use the numbers to figure out how the produce you are buying has been grown. A sticker with four digits means the food was conventionally grown. Five digits starting with an eight indicates genetically engineered produce. Five digits starting with a nine means the food was organically grown.

Fruits and vegetables:

For the ladies, eat plenty of fruits and veggies during your menstrual cycle. These naturally cleanse the body. Many vegetables are high in calcium, magnesium, and potassium, which help relieve and prevent muscle spasms during your period. Fruits are an excellent source of natural anti-inflammatory substances, like bioflavonoids and vitamin C. These nutrients not only strengthen the blood vessels that aid circulation to areas of muscle tension in the pelvis but also reduce the pain from menstrual cramps through their anti-inflammatory effect.

By upping your consumption of green vegetables, you can help avoid calcium deficiency and prevent menstrual cramps. Complex carbohydrates, such as whole grains, fresh fruit, and vegetables may also help relieve premenstrual symptoms. You may want to back off of animal protein for a few days leading up to the start of your period, and go more for complex carbs instead.

Nuts: 2–3 servings daily of raw nuts, not roasted

(When you roast nuts, they become rancid and hydrogenated and can cause cancer.)

Some examples would be almonds, pecans, cashews, Brazil nuts, walnuts, chestnuts, filberts, acorns, and pine nuts.

To you it shall be your food. Originally, the green herbs were given by God as food for the animals in Genesis 1:30. The word "shall" here *is a command, not a suggestion.* The Lord is telling us we have no option when it comes to eating whole grains, fresh fruits, vegetables, raw nuts, and raw seeds . . . Five is fine, but nine is divine!

"And to every beast of the earth, and to every fowl of the air and to everything that creepeth upon the earth, I have given every green herb for meat and it was so."

These green herbs were added to man's diet after he sinned (to help fight disease) and are a part of our diet today.

There's something truly unique about the nourishment you get from eating leafy green vegetables like broccoli, kale, and spinach (preferably raw and organic).

Nature gives us another potent class of greens like rosemary and curcumin, sea vegetables like spirulina and ecklonia, and long grasses like barley and rye. These foods create a wave of pure nutrition surging through your entire body, carrying potent free-radical fighters and high-level detoxifiers to each and every cell of your body. These leave you feeling completely cleansed, vibrant, and healthy.

Most of us struggle to eat one or two servings a day of basic green vegetables. Sometimes, it is even hard to find these classes of food today, and that is where supplementation is necessary. You can read all about supplements in a later chapter.

Some of these vegetables include:
Leafy herbs:
- Celery
- Cabbage
- Kale
- Chard
- Lettuce, etc.

Flowers:
- Cauliflower
- Broccoli
- Artichoke

Roots:
- Carrots
- Beets
- Potatoes
- Turnips, etc.

****These foods are your key to total health****

The cultures living long on the earth eat these foods.

Why are these foods so special? It's all about living foods—raw foods—because of the nutrition and life gives life; when you cook foods, they are dead; 50 percent of the nutrition is destroyed. Raw foods give more energy; the digestive enzymes are lost when food is cooked over 118 degrees . . . the vitamin C is destroyed and the B vitamins are nearly annihilated. Sometimes, 75 percent of the nutrition is destroyed by processed foods (by refining and preservatives).

Oxygen is the key. Addison's disease is the atrophy of the adrenal glands. Raw foods and raw food supplements are the key.

The most vital nutrients to all cells are those that provide oxygen. Cancer cells cannot grow where oxygen exists. All degenerative disease grows and proliferates where the cells don't get any or enough oxygen.

The last chapter in the Bible (Revelation 22:2) deals with the leaves for the healing of the nations.

I love the example in Daniel 1: 8-16. The story is told of a ten-day trial of eating vegetables and drinking water instead of the king's rich food (that diet would be comparable to the SAD, the standard American diet). After this test period, we are told Daniel and his three friends were judged to be better in appearance and smarter than those who had eaten the rich foods. Some could interpret that to mean we are to only eat a vegetarian diet, but the point is to expose a contrast between unhealthful food practices of that day to a more simple diet and its benefits.

We too practice unhealthful food choices. Sadly, the majority of people living in America will suffer the consequences of a poor diet, which often leads to premature death.

But we can change that. We have God's power, and He can change our taste buds. *It's time for us to start eating a diet of prevention and not waiting until it is too late.* I spoke with a precious woman the other day and she was crying because her twenty-five-year-old brother is dying of leukemia. What if her brother had known how to eat to not get cancer? I can assure you that his life would have been completely different. He has a wife and three little children.

What can you do to protect your own health? As much as possible, eat plant-based foods that are fresh, whole, unprocessed, and organically grown. Eat as many of these foods as possible, and try to eat them raw. Cooking damages the nutrient content of our foods (and that would especially be microwave cooking). Healthy populations eat about 80 percent of their diets raw. This may sound difficult at first, but it actually becomes easier than having to cook meals. Eat more fresh salads and fresh fruits. You don't have to make these changes overnight. Attack this like a worm attacks an apple, one bite at a time! Find one new concept, and work with that for a couple of weeks. Once proficient, then work on changing something else.

When we cook foods, we destroy up to 85 percent of the nutrients. And the cooking can denature the protein molecules and turn them into chemicals that are known to be toxic and even carcinogenic (cancer causing). Eating raw foods is the way to go, and eating a diet that is about 80 percent raw is what you should strive for.

Processing of foods includes anything that happens to the food before you eat it. The more that happens to it, the more nutrition is lost and the more likely toxic contaminants have been added. This would usually be foods that come in jars, cans, and packages. More than 50 percent of the average American's diet consists of processed foods. Dr. Colin Campbell of Cornell University did a study on the health effects of diets in sixty-five different Chinese provinces. His conclusion is that the closer one approaches a total plant food diet, the greater the benefits. And this was the original health plan mandate given to us by God in the beginning. The average American diet, however, consists of 37 percent of its calories coming from fat. In China, the fat intake varies from 6 percent up to 24 percent, with an average of 14 percent. The healthiest people consumed the least amount of fat. Many prestigious medical journals confirm that a high fat diet is a high-risk dietary factor for colon, prostate, and breast cancer.

Protein intake is also lower in China. In China, about 10 percent of dietary protein comes from animal sources. Whereas in the United States, it's about 70 percent. The China study found that the type of protein consumed had a huge effect on health. Even as little as 20 percent of animal protein will increase cholesterol levels in the blood, and high cholesterol has a clear relationship to chronic diseases such as cancer, heart disease, etc. Animal protein is chemically different from plant protein, and this difference can exhibit very undesirable effects. Remember when God added a little bit of animal protein to our diet and gave us permission to eat that little bit, the ages of the patriarchs began to decline. Eating a lot of meat can be dangerous! We'll delve into this more deeply in the next chapter.

The conclusion we can make from all of this is that the best diet for everyone is one based on a variety of fresh, mostly uncooked, organically grown high-quality plant-based foods. This diet has the greatest possibility of supplying your cells with all the nutrients they need. Eating a high fat diet of animal protein will interfere with the successful operation of those cells.

Each year the Environmental Working Group identifies its "Dirty Dozen." These are the twelve fruits and vegetables that contain the highest amount of pesticides, and thus, should be purchased as organic whenever possible.

The "Dirty Dozen" are as follows:
- Celery
- Peaches
- Strawberries
- Sweet bell peppers
- Nectarines
- Strawberries
- Grapes
- Spinach
- Lettuce
- Cucumbers
- Blueberries
- Potatoes

Whether you buy organic or conventional produce, I recommend you wash it with a surfactant to remove herbicides, chemicals, and pesticides and just for general cleanliness overall.

We offer this cleaner from our office. To order, call (972) 380-5363.

CHAPTER 6

Foods That Kill: (Avoid As If Your Life Depends on It)

What's in God's Garbage Can?

What's in God's garbage can? Friend or foe?

Did you know Americans eat a million animals an hour and 150 pounds of refined sugar a year?

Wow! That's a lot of animals and a lot of sugar. Is it really good for us?

What blocks the delivery of oxygen to the cells and organs? When people follow a diet of high fat content, concentrated sugars, and too much alcohol, triglycerides reach high levels in the blood and cause red blood cells to clump together. Clumped red blood cells are less capable of carrying oxygen, and they clog the capillaries, diminishing the ability to get life-sustaining oxygen to the living cells of the body. This particularly affects the brain, the carotid arteries, liver, and kidneys. When cells of the body do not receive adequate oxygen, they cannot function optimally; this leads to decreased endurance, sluggishness, poor memory, and strokes. Partial oxygen starvation produces degenerative diseases: heart disease, diabetes, atherosclerosis, gall bladder issues, erectile dysfunction, cancer, etc. The body begins to degenerate. With poor nutritional habits, degeneration usually begins by age forty and is in evidence by age fifty. The sad thing is that the next several decades of life will be spent in doctor's offices and hospitals, having operations, taking medications, and paying the pharmaceutical companies a lot of your hard-earned money instead of enjoying retirement or life in general. And it will decrease the inheritance you could have left to your children and grandchildren. This is the three score and ten, which is considered to be a curse. Eating right and taking the right kind of supplements is a lot better and much more fun. And it's a whole lot less expensive.

For our health's sake, our staples should be fresh fruits, vegetables, and whole grains. It doesn't mean that we can't eat any meat, fish, or fowl, but He gave us guidelines on which ones will make us sick and which we can eat just a little bit of. He gives us permission to eat just a little bit of clean meat but admonishes us to never eat the unclean meat for all the generations to come. The point is that Americans eat too much meat, and often, it is the wrong kind. This fact alone contributes to why we are so sick with long and lingering illnesses.

Leviticus 3:17 says, "It shall be a statute forever throughout all your generations and in all your dwelling places that you eat neither fat nor blood." Today, both the American Medical Association and the World Health Organization say that the cause of hardening of the arteries, all heart disease, and cancer are directly related to the fact that we eat too much fat. Now, it's interesting that there is no fat or cholesterol in plant foods and vegetation. And there is no fiber in meat and dairy.

Clean and Unclean Animals

God created clean and unclean animals. *Why did He make a distinction?* After the flood, the vegetation was affected to some degree, and God introduced a little bit of clean animal protein. He did not command man to eat meat, but merely gave permission to add a little bit of clean animal protein. It was intended mainly for the celebrations, not as a daily staple.

Eating today's red meat is linked to fifty thousand deaths annually in our nation. Of course, the Cattlemen's Association is not advertising that. The food group we call meat and dairy contributes to 90 percent of all physical problems we are experiencing. I'm not suggesting that you can never eat meat, but statistics are telling and should not be ignored.

*The clean animals God told us we could eat **are vegetarian animals.*** Isn't that interesting? The unclean animals eat ***dead, diseased animals.*** That is their purpose. They are garbage collectors. He gave us the clean and the unclean in the air, land, and in the waters. He gave us permission to eat only a little bit of the clean animals. He warned us about eating the unclean, saying they were not food for us. They are His garbage collectors and scavengers. He has not changed the anatomy of the unclean; it's still the same. He has not changed the anatomy of man to accommodate eating the unclean. Had he not created His garbage collectors in the air, the land, and the waters, disease would proliferate and mankind would die off. The unclean had a specific purpose. He said, "My children for all the generations to come, do not eat the unclean animals or they will be an abomination to you." He says it over and over again. What is cancer, heart disease, diabetes, and arthritis? Are these diseases a blessing or an abomination? If they are a blessing, we should pray for everyone to get these diseases. Would all the generations to come be just for the Old Testament or just for the nation of Israel? I don't think so. We are a very important generation.

When we add meat to our diets, we are adding purines and many other bacterial toxins to our bloodstream. Meat adds too concentrated of a protein source with nasty, waxy fats, which lodge in our bodies, only to rear their ugly heads and cloud the blood, lymph, and mind—not to mention the colon.

Conversely, eating a diet rich in super greens, sprouted grains, and other plant-based foods does not do this. Plant foods do not have cholesterol, but they are rich in fiber, enzymes, and antioxidants. Animals, however, do not have fiber, antioxidants, and enzymes that prevent our top killers.

Let's Look at Some Guidelines Now Pertaining to Eating Meat

It's interesting to note that this post-deluvian (after the flood) permission to eat even the clean animals produced a phenomenon. Almost immediately, the life span of the human race fell from around 800 to about 150 years. The flood experience also demolishes a popular argument used by those who insist on eating both clean and unclean animals. Some claim that the law of unclean foods applied only to the Jewish people. This cannot be correct, since there were no Jews in Noah's day when the restriction was laid out by God himself. Furthermore, the Bible declares that the forbidden–meat law will still be in effect at the second coming of Jesus (Isaiah 66: 15-17).

There are meats that our Chief Nutritionist gave us for the grocery list, and there are also animals that He said would be an abomination to us if eaten—not to Him, but to us.

I don't want something in my life that is an abomination, do you?

I think it's curious that when God gave the command in Genesis regarding what to eat, it was a command to eat fresh fruits and vegetables. But when it comes to meat, He gives us permission to eat only a little bit—but it is not a command; it is only "permissible."

Leviticus 3:17: "This shall be a perpetual statute throughout your generations in all your dwellings: You shall eat neither fat nor blood."

God's harshest words were spoken about the third major food group. Why would this be?

Dr. Gordon Tessler says, "When you walk by a steak house or a fast food restaurant, what do you smell? You smell the aroma of burning fat and that smell draws—or a better word is *seduces*—millions to buy hamburgers, French fries, and then there are hot donuts that are soaked with rancid oil, which causes breast, colon, and prostate cancer." The burning of animal fat is the "sweet aroma" for anyone who has smelled a sizzling steak as it cooks over mesquite wood or barbequed ribs or bacon crackling in the frying pan. But according to the Lord, all fat belongs to Him on the altar and is not be to be eaten (Leviticus 3:17). He repeats this several times; we should not ignore it.

Leviticus 7:23: "Speak to the children of Israel, saying: 'You shall not eat any fat of the ox, sheep, or goat." The next verse says, "And the fat of a beast that dies naturally, and the fat of what is torn by wild animals, may be used in any other way, but you shall by **no means** eat it." And again in verses 25 and 26, God is repeating this over and over.

It's interesting that the American Heart Association, the American Medical Association, and the American Cancer Association have spent trillions of dollars of our tax money in the last forty-plus years trying to figure out what is causing these diseases, only to find out why heart disease is the number one killer, cancer the number two killer, and diabetes the third. All of these prestigious organizations have come to the realization that there is only one thing that is the main underlying cause of all these problems, and that is that Americans eat too much fat. Eating a million animals an hour can contribute to that!

The average American eats 50-60 percent of his diet in saturated fat. We know that if you eat fat, it accumulates in your body, and animal fat causes heart disease and cancer. All of these big organizations are now saying, "Cut down on saturated fat," but God said it four thousand years ago! Medical science is always having to catch up with God's Word!

We know that the life is in the blood, so it follows that disease is also in the blood. Here's a little tip on removing blood from red meat:

Soak the red meat in water for fifteen minutes, then salt it. Add water and soak for one hour. This will not change the flavor, but it removes the blood.

For years, we have ranked number two in the world in our incidence of heart attacks. Hardening of the arteries is the basic cause. The only place that tops us is a country in Eastern Finland. It's also curious that we have ranked consistently number two in the world in our fat intake. Do you believe God meant what He was saying in the Old Testament?

I have heard people call this legalism—that they're not under the law. Let me just say our bodies have not yet been redeemed. They have not yet been glorified. Whether you think you are under a law or not, you have the optic nerve, the pancreatic system, and the lymphatic system; these are all physical, and they function well on good nutrients, and that is a law!

We are not talking laws for salvation but that it may go well with us on the earth—so that we are walking in blessing and not cursing. It doesn't mean that you won't go to heaven if you eat the hog or shellfish, but it does mean that you most likely will get there more quickly. And that is exactly what is happening in the body of Christ. Yet many are eating these foods in the name of grace, and it isn't working. Paul says, "Shall we continue to do wrong that grace may abound?" (Romans 6:1).

God Addresses the Food Group Americans Call Meat and Dairy

Let's look at Leviticus 11:1. This is one of the main passages dealing with clean and unclean foods. The chapter starts out talking to the Israelites, and sometimes people argue that we are not Israel. But I believe that we have been engrafted into the olive tree. Our hearts have been circumcised in the new covenant; the laws of God have been written on our hearts; we can receive the same blessings promised to the Israelites (Galatians 3).

God gave us a system so we can quickly tell which animals are clean. These animals He names, including the ox, calf, steer, sheep, and buffalo, all are vegetarian. They completely process foods; they have two or three stomachs and get rid of their poisons within twenty-four hours, so they are truly clean in the sense of their digestive tracks.

Leviticus 11:1 has to do with clean and unclean animals. And verses 2-4 go on to say, "These are the beasts which you shall eat among all the beasts that are on the earth. Whatsoever parteth the hoof, and is cloven footed, and chews the cud, among the beasts, that ye shall eat. These shall ye not eat of them that chew the cud, or of them that divide the hoof: as the camel, because he chews the cud but does not divide the hoof, he is unclean to you."

Verses 7-8 then speak to one of America's favorite delicacies: "And the swine [pig], though he divides the hoof and be cloven footed, yet he chews not the cud: he is unclean to you. Of their flesh shall ye not eat, and their carcass shall you not touch; they are unclean to you."

One of the top foods I tell all my clients not to eat is anything from the pig. That includes cold cuts, pepperoni, hot dogs, luncheon meats, sausage, bacon (which is the number one carcinogenic meat in our nation), and ham (the most unholy meat served on Easter, the most holy day of the year).

I admonish Christian leaders and all pastors to take leadership in this area. When you have gatherings for children's ministry, do not serve hot dogs. Don't condone serving your flock foods God said were an abomination for all the generations to come. When you set up Christian retreats, advise conference leaders to forgo sausage, bacon, ham sandwiches, hot dogs, or pigs in a blanket on the menu. They may be tiny and small, but they are filled with disease. Is that what you want to offer your church members? While you may be doing seminars on healing, you are not setting a biblical example and model of how to walk in health. If we are walking in health, we won't need instantaneous healing. Most conference organizers are not knowledgeable and serve the food of the world. It's time to begin taking leadership in this area of the Christian life—body, soul, and spirit (I Thessalonians 5:23).

In Deuteronomy, God tells us, His children, to never eat certain meats because if we do, we will have long, lingering, and painful illnesses. Was this just for the Old Testament? No. He says over and over again, for all the generations to come, don't eat them because they will be an abomination to you. If you know scientifically what pork and shellfish products do to your body, you most likely will not continue to put them into your temple. It's a choice.

The manufacturers of cold cuts, bacon, etc., do not bother to tell you that sodium nitrite has been clinically proven to cause a 6,700 percent increase in pancreatic cancer. It also produces a compound called nitrosamines in the stomach, which are one of the most effective agents known to man for causing malignant brain tumors in laboratory animals and contribute to stomach and pancreatic cancer in humans.

If we have this knowledge, why in the world do we feed these foods to our families? It is for lack of knowledge that God's people are perishing. We are not victims. Our bodies are the temple of the Holy Spirit. We need to take care of them to fulfill the very call of God on our lives—that is our very purpose in being here. Or would you rather be wasting away at the hospital? *I know you wouldn't!*

Hogs, Swine, Pigs . . . Do You Like to Eat a Pig?

Let's focus on pigs for a minute—a church favorite. Pigs are the filthiest of all animals.

Americans call these animals hot dogs, pepperoni, honey baked ham, pork loin, bacon (the number one cancer-causing meat in the world), sausage, and more . . .

Let's talk about one of America's favorites . . . HOT DOGS!

Children who eat twelve or more hot dogs a month are 9.5 times more likely to get leukemia (the number one killer of children next to accidents). When a pregnant mother eats hot dogs during pregnancy, the incidence of brain cancer in her children increases dramatically as well.

The average person consumes fifty of them per year. Hot dogs are one of the most nutritionally bankrupt, cancer causing-foods in the world. According to the American Institute for Cancer Research (AICR), eating just one hot dog raises your risk for colorectal cancer by 21 percent. Americans spend $2.5 billion on hot dogs in the US supermarkets, which amounts to more than one billion packages of wieners. During peak hot dog season—Memorial Day to Labor Day —Americans belt down seven billion dogs.

On the Fourth of July alone, Americans consume 150 million hot dogs—enough to stretch from Washington, DC, to Los Angeles more than five times! Most of the meat and meat by-products come from confined animal feeding operations (CAFOs) where animals are tortured in crowded, unhealthy, unsanitary, and cruel conditions, as the primary goal is cheap food, not quality food.

I've heard people who raise pigs say that if they don't keep their eye on a pig to feed them the right thing, those pigs will go off and eat anything. If there is an animal with tumors and cancer, they will go off and eat it. Pigs carry over two hundred known diseases. They have more arthritis than any other animal. It is my opinion that a person can eat a pig, and the arthritis from the pig is transferred to the person. Pigs have up to two hundred different worms and nineteen parasites, including trichinae. We lead the world in trichinosis, and these parasites are not cooked away because they are involved inside the body. Biologically, pigs have not changed in 3,500 years. God has not changed our anatomies nor has he changed the anatomy of the unclean animals to allow us to safely eat them. So whatever you want to believe about not being under a law is up to you, but it is a law that has not been changed to accommodate us for health and we have not changed and that is a law we dare not break. A pig is cloven footed and if you squeeze on their legs, a green goo (green is usually a sign of health, but not in this case) that oozes out of their feet. This is how their bodies excrete. You can take a dead rat filled with maggots, and the pig will eat the whole thing. If you want good health, don't eat the pig. I can guarantee you that if you eat the pepperoni, the sausage, the bacon, and the ham, you will not have good health. I can also guarantee you that if you eat the shrimp, lobster, catfish, clams, and crab, you will not have good health. God said it and I believe it when He said that if you eat them, it will be an abomination to you. When you eat the clam chowder, as delicious as it may be, it is no different than eating roach chowder or rat chowder. God instructed us to not defile this body; it is holy and set apart unto the Lord.

I hear people say hogs are not what they used to be. Now we have them in "nice" pens, and they are kept in buildings. But did you know that every year in hog buildings they have to change the hardware on the doors because of the stench that comes off these unclean animals? The hog carries a lot of respiratory problems, and many hog producers have respiratory and lung issues too. If you do have respiratory problems, I ask you if you, too, have been eating the sausage, pepperoni, honey baked ham, or cold cuts. If so, there may be a connection with your condition. The good news is that we can do something about that. Sometimes, it can be just little changes that can make a huge difference.

The hog is omnivorous, which is an animal that eats animals and plants. When you eat an animal, you are eating all the diseases and parasites of that animal. They are coming right into your system, so God said, "Don't eat them, and eat only the animals that only eat plants because they are the clean animals to eat."

Pork and other unclean meats normally contain a high parasite infestation, and these meats digest too quickly for the human metabolism, thereby causing a rapid rise in blood ureas. This overloads the system and may cause excessive stress on the heart and other elimination organs. Think about what animal God sent the demons into.

Why is an animal with hoofs that are not divided not clean? Just think about yourself. If you don't take a bath and change your socks, and you wear your shoes for twenty-four hours, your feet begin to smell. Have you ever sat near someone who had stinky feet? It's awful, isn't it? The poisons of your body go down into your feet and into your socks and as that perspiration comes out, it goes into your shoes.

What do you think about something that has no way of releasing the poison—like a hoofed animal? But a cloven-hoofed animal has a way to expel the perspiration and the poison from its body. And so if you eat that kind of animal you get less poison than with a hoofed animal.

Animals that chew the cud have more than one stomach. By the time they totally chew their food and it gets into the intestines, it is very easily digested, so that animal is going to have healthier flesh because his digestive system is better.

The clean animals (which eat only vegetables . . . not diseased animals) that chew the cud and have a divided hoof are the ox, sheep, goat, deer, cow, steer, buffalo, etc. Because of the sacculated condition of the alimentary canal and the secondary cud receptacle, these animals practically have three stomachs as refining agencies and cleansing laboratories for purifying their food. This cleanses the system of all poisonous and deleterious matter. It takes their clean vegetable food over twenty-four hours to be turned into flesh, which even the pre-mosaic law said was clean. This was not mere "ceremonial" cleansing, but it was made hygienically and physiologically clean and whole-some.

In comparison, we find that the swine's anatomy, as a supplement to his bad appetite, has but one poorly constructed stomach arrangement and very limited excretory organs. Consequently, in about four hours after the pig has eaten his polluted swill and other putrid, offensive matter, man may eat the same second-handed putrid, offensive matter off the ribs of the pig. *Think twice before you eat the next barbecued pork sandwich.*

What Happens When We Eat Unclean Flesh?

You have an almost immediate rise in blood ureas, which means the food is being digested too quickly and the body cannot assimilate it. It causes the blood protein to go up too fast, increases viscosity of the blood and blood pressure, heightens the strength of heart beat, and also hastens aging.

It's curious that all unclean meat does this, and the clean meat does not. This is not a coincidence. But it's also curious that the foods God told us we could eat promote health. They normalize triglycerides and glands, stabilize blood sugar, and provide oxygen in the cells.

Conversely, the unclean animals are meat-eating animals that clean up anything that is left dead in the sky, the land, and the waters. If a dog (or any animal whatsoever) should die in the field and lie in the sun and bloat until it is broken open and the maggots and putrefaction have set in, then the swine or other scavengers will come and eat up all the filth and putrid matter, thereby keeping disease germs from spreading all over the earth and killing off mankind. But scavengers were never created for human consumption. They are God's garbage collectors.

Swine, by its very nature, is poisonous, deadly, and diseased. The flesh of the swine is said by many authorities to be the prime cause of much of our ill health in America. Eating the hog causes blood diseases, weakness of the stomach, liver troubles, eczema, consumption, tumors, lung conditions, stomach and pancreatic cancer, etc. The trichinae is one of the eighteen or nineteen worms found in hogs, not to mention lice or other diseases such as rickets, thumps, mange, etc. The trichinae worm is deadly. A single bite of infected pork can cripple or condemn the victim to a lifetime of aches and pains. For this unique disease, trichinosis, there is no sure cure. Have you ever cooked a pork egg roll in a microwave? Microwaves cook unevenly, so you may be eating uncooked pork.

You may see the words "US Government Inspected and Passed" stamped on a package of pork. Those words do not mean that any official inspection has been made as to whether this pork has trichinosis or not. It has merely passed the routine inspection given meat in general (regulations as of 1976).

Dr. Maurice Hall, as chief of the Division of Zoology of the US Public Health Service, commented, "It appears to be a legitimate demand that when a man exchanged dollars for pork, he should not do it on the basis that he may be purchasing his 'death warrant' speaking in regard to the infected meat of the swine. Physicians have confused trichinosis with some fifty ailments, ranging from typhoid fever to acute alcoholism."

"That pain in your arm or leg may be arthritis or rheumatism, but it may be trichinosis; that pain in your back may be a gall bladder involvement, but it may mean trichinosis," says Senator Thomas C. Desmond, who served as chairman of the New York Trichinosis Commission.

Can't Cook It Out:
Parasites, Worms, and Disease—Still Kickin'!

A university lab heated trichinae-laden swine flesh to an unbelievably high temperature and then viewed it under a microscope. To the amazement of the technicians, some worms were still alive and moving about. The supposition that all of these worms can be killed through cooking is not to be relied upon. And this was after cooking it at 500 degrees. Why take a chance with such a crippler and killer? And we know what Jesus thought about the pork. He cast the demons into the pigs. If we know what Jesus thought about the pig, I think we should definitely stay away from it. If you have eaten pork, you have eaten parasites. Those parasites were still alive even after cooking pork on the grill at 500 degrees. But even if you have eaten pork and the parasites were dead, who wants to eat dead parasites and have them in your blood stream and intestines?

The trichinae are just one worm found in the swine. Others include a large round kidney worm (which can be as long as eighteen inches), the gullet worm, and three kinds of stomach worms—a tiny hair worm, a hookworm, and the thorn-headed worm—in the small intestine. There are several species of nodular worms and one species of whip worm in the large intestine (Drs. Hess and Clark in *The Barnyard Doctor*).

Peter Wina, chief of pathobiology at the Walter Reid Army Institute of Research, says, "We have a tremendous parasite problem right here in America, but it's just not being addressed." Now, obviously, we have the best of medicine in the entire world, but when we go see a doctor, he rarely thinks to look for parasites first.

Dr. Hazel Parcels states that "Eighty-five percent of adult North Americans are infected with parasites."

But perhaps the most surprising statement comes from Dr. Frank Nova, chief of the Laboratory for Parasitic Diseases at the National Institute of Health, when he says, "In terms of numbers, there are more parasitic infections acquired in this country than in Africa."

To sum up this section, let's take a quick peek at the meats we can eat a little bit of and the meats we should never eat, according to God.

Clean = beef, lamb, mutton, veal

Unclean = pork, dog, cat, rabbit or rat, cat, horse, or mule

With regard to seafood, Leviticus 11:9-12 says, "***When we eat them, they must have fins and scales.***"

I had a young woman in my office who said, "Lilli, I think I can give up the pepperoni, sausage, and bacon, but shrimp? I love shrimp." She said it with such passion. I said, "I understand, I used to love shrimp, too, until I learned what that shrimp just ate for dinner."

That shrimp just ate the excrement of all the fish above and cleaned up the waters of all the dead, diseased fish. And that is good in its place (I Timothy 4:4), but it was never intended to be on plates. Shrimp are garbage collectors for God's children. God told us that if we eat the shellfish (for all the generations to come), we would be very sick. And in the Christian community and in our nation at large, we are very sick, and most people love shrimp and lobster. And sadly, most think it is healthy. And most nutrition books have recipes for it. But God has the final word, and He said do not eat it. It was not created for you to eat.

What Is the Purpose of Fins and Scales?

Fins enable the fish to move along in the waters; scales are there to protect. If a fish has fins, and if it is in a polluted area, he instinctively knows to swim out of it—and he will. The scales protect the fish and keep out infection and disease. If a fish has a broken scale or does not have scales, it is an unhealthy source of fish.

Let's take a quick peak at some examples of the clean fish God told us we can eat.

Clean: Haddock, salmon, sole, sea bass, halibut, cod, sea trout, and grouper

Unclean: Catfish, shrimp, lobster, clams, oysters, scallops, and crabs are some.

You are not under the law for salvation, but the laws of what to eat or not eat have not changed if you want to walk in health. This is a dietary law that is just as relevant today as ever—just as the law of gravity is still in effect.

Sometimes people ask why these are unclean.

The unclean fish are scavengers. That means they clean up the dead, diseased fish in the waters, and they eat the excrement of all the other fish above. They are bottom feeders. Shellfish quite often have extremely high levels of toxic materials and parasites; there have been reports of people dying from eating shellfish. We must remember that shellfish are in the water for one purpose and that is to eat the debris and eliminated waste of other fish. The shrimp, for example, eat the excrement of the fish above and this is good in its place (1 Timothy 4:4), but they are obviously not meant to be on our plates. Do we really need to be putting this kind of filth and garbage in our cells and bloodstream?

Isn't it interesting that the fish God told us to eat is healing to the body? (Eskimoes, for example, do not suffer from heart disease.)

These good fish contain EPA and DHA, the essential omegas that prevent strokes and heart attacks, lower blood pressure, take the swelling out of joints, relieve migraine headaches, and help with skin problems like psoriasis, to name just a few.

Let's look at Leviticus 11:13-21. Good: Chickens, turkeys, geese, ducks, doves, quail, Cornish hen, etc.

Some birds are bloodsuckers, like vultures; they eat dead things. The eagle, the ostrich, etc. are also unclean.

Consider Leviticus 11:27. Animals that go on paws like lions and tigers: padded feet are vulnerable to disease, so they take poison into them and they don't chew their cuds; they don't have cloven hoofs and they feed on humans.

Leviticus 11:29: These also are unclean: the mouse, the weasel, the lizard, and other creeping things—they are scavengers. Don't touch them while they are alive or dead. They go in areas where there is disease and infected things and their fur and their skin carry it, and when you touch it, it can infect you.

The bubonic plague, which killed millions of people in Europe, was basically brought on by rats. They would crawl into places, and in some way, they would get to the people, and people would touch them, and they would be infected.

Why did He give us these better health laws? He taught these in the wilderness to the people who were going into the Promised Land.

But what if you go into the Promised Land *(or your long antici-pated retirement days), and you don't live very long to enjoy it?* And even today, for people who are living under the curse of three score and ten, many have hoped to enjoy their retirement days and travel and enjoy so many wonders of the world but find that their health is failing them. The body, which runs on good nutrition, is now break-ing down and dying because we have failed to tend to it the way God intended.

People who lived in Canaan just ate anything. They ate blood, rats, dogs, cats, creeping things, etc. After reviewing Canaanite civilization records, researchers found that the Canaanites had a very short lifespan because of the way they lived. Do you think God likes it when you are sick? To those going into the Promised Land, he said, "I am giving you farms that you never farmed, trees you never planted, wells you did not dig, animals that never belonged to you, and I am going to give you a land flowing with milk and honey, but when you get in, I want you to live long in that land." And the way you live long is to keep these ways of eating. He fed them manna (which is a seed like coriander) in the wilderness for almost forty years, and they were not sick and they were not weak; their feet did not swell. Why? Because they ate what God fed them.

Meat contains white fat. An average American meat-eater puts over eighty-five pounds of fat (cholesterol) into his or her body each year. This fat clogs the arteries, which ultimately is the cause of heart attacks and strokes that will kill approximately 50 percent of our population. We are told that we need meat for protein and strength. Do you know what a cow eats for protein? He eats grass and alfalfa. And do they usually grow very strong? There is more protein in our alfalfa tablets than there is in beef. But when I say the word protein to Americans, they invariably think animal protein. That is not so with people in countries who are living long and well.

Other Unhealthy Food Choices

What about cow's milk? This is a tender subject . . .

According to the USDA the average American consumes 630 pounds of milk, yogurt, and ice cream per year.

Do you have cow's milk in your refrigerator? Why are you and your family drinking milk from the cow?

We've been duped; it is not for kids or adults. *Milk is for newborns.* And cow's milk is for a newborn calf. Have we not been weaned from our mother's milk?

Note all of the advertising for drinking cow's milk revolves around calcium. *We do not assimilate calcium from milk.* When I mention how unhealthy drinking cow's milk is, I am frequently asked why the

Bible talks about a land flowing with milk and honey. The biblical definition for "milk and honey" is a metaphor meaning all good things. God's blessings and the Promised Land must have been referred to as a land of extraordinary fertility. The phrase "flowing with milk and honey" is understood to be hyperbolically descriptive of the land's richness; hence, its current use is to express the overflow of pure abundance.

Cow's milk is another food from and of the world's system. It is causing all kinds of disease in America. It is a processed food, as it undergoes a process called *pasteurization*. This changes the complete chemical state of the milk. It changes it so much that when experimental animals are given cow's milk, they all get sick and die. Raw, fresh from the cow, cow's milk is for baby calves to grow big and strong fast. Give a baby calf cow's pasteurized milk, and it dies within two months. This should cause concern about our extensive intake of milk. Practically every client whom I interview has cow's milk in his or her refrigerator, and most think it is a healthy staple for our diets. Milk is for newborns; it is not intended for human adults. God gave every newborn nourishment from that mommy species. Most of us old enough to read this book have been weaned from mommies' milk. Milk, by God's design, is for a newborn. As adults, we simply do not need milk. And we certainly do not assimilate calcium from cow's milk.

About 80 percent of the average person's pesticide load comes from eating animal meat and dairy. Simply stop eating these foods, and you can cut out 80 percent of your pesticide load! Where do you think our children are picking up all those carcinogens? It's mostly from eating meat and dairy. The pesticides and other agricultural chemicals on the grains fed to our farm animals accumulate in their fatty tissues. And then they are passed on to us through the dairy and the meat. These are some of the reasons why I don't recommend dairy. Animal meat should always be grass-fed, free of hormones and antibiotics. Dairy is a very poor source of nutrients, yet a good source of toxins, thus giving us a powerful combination of deficiency and toxicity. Americans eat more dairy than the rest of the world combined, and this contributes to all disease in our nation.

I remember the four food groups that were posted on the board in elementary school. I thought they were kind of like the Ten Commandments until I found out that the Dairy Council had put them there. And you can imagine what that means . . . HUGE PROFITS AT OUR EXPENSE.

What about you? Do you have cow's milk in your refrigerator? If so, why are you drinking milk from another species? There is nothing in milk that is good for people. We don't get calcium from milk. Yes, there is calcium in milk, but to assimilate calcium, you have to have an enzyme for the mineral to hang onto. Because of the processing of milk, the enzymes have been destroyed.

Do you know any children who have had tubes in their ears? Cow's milk is the culprit.

Do you know anyone who suffers with asthma, allergies, or sinus issues? Cow's milk is a huge contributing factor. Why do you think practically everyone in America is drinking milk? There is only one reason and that is because we have been brainwashed by the Dairy Council. The Dairy Council has been around since around 1915, and they started their heavy campaigning in the 1950s. Their platform revolved around drinking cow's milk for healthy bones and teeth. Is it curious to you that we are the only nation that cross-species when it comes to milk, and we have more unhealthy bones and teeth than any other nation? We have more osteopenia and osteoporosis than any other country. More women die from hip fractures in the US than they do of breast cancer. Americans are 6 percent of the world's population, yet we drink more milk than the other 94 percent combined. You would think that Americans would have the strongest bones in the world, but we don't. Instead, we have the highest osteoporosis rates in the world. The cultures that do not drink any milk do not have osteoporosis.

We think milk is just milk, but the FDA adds up to eighty-two drugs to cow's milk in the production of dairy products.

We are the only nation (maybe there's one other) that cross-species when it comes to milk. It contains all sorts of proteins in it that are harmful to humans. It is not good for our hearts, bones, or respiratory system. It was simply not intended for humans. Again, it is the number one cause of allergies, sinus problems, and many respiratory conditions. It causes mucous, which impedes and blocks healing. What you have been told your entire life about milk is simply a lie. Your glass of milk, even the low fat variety, is awash in fat (the equivalent of three slices of bacon), cholesterol, antibiotics, bacteria, and the most distasteful ingredient—pus!

Well-meaning nutritionists reiterate that we need the calcium found in milk and dairy to keep our bones strong. How is that concept working for us? Celebrities pose with milk mustaches. It is time for us to stop being in denial about the foods and drinks that are making us and our children sick. I'll bet you agree!

This is a very tender subject for many people until they realize, sadly, what it is doing to their bodies. A well-known pediatrician says that cow's milk is a food for big animals with little tiny brains. He is very well thought of, and his position is, "get your kids off cow's milk." Milk is highly allergenic and the main cause of ear infections and the need for tubes in the ears.

In Nature, No Animal Pasteurizes Its Milk

Cow's milk is one of the most dangerous substances we can put in our body. We are told milk is the perfect food and needed for calcium. What we are not told is that milk is a processed food that has been pasteurized and heated to at least 160 degrees. This changes the calcium to an inorganic form, which cannot be assimilated by the body. *In nature no animal pasteurizes its milk.* And no animal or mammal drinks the milk of another species, nor does it ever drink milk after the age of weaning. The only source of bad cholesterol (LDL) comes from animal products. Animal products are just not the best food. (Remember Genesis 1:29, 30.) Better sources of calcium would be found in cantaloupe and raw almonds. Almonds have twice the amount of calcium than raw milk. Today, we need to supplement with calcium, but it must be the right kind. There are many calcium supplements that are going straight through people, and some calcium supplements are the main cause of kidney stones.

Healthier sources of milk for making our protein smoothies would be almond, hazelnut, or rice milk. These are not dairy. Do not drink soy milk. We must supplement with good organic calcium supplements. But they must be the right kind, as inorganic calcium supplements do go straight through you.

Milk and the Cancer Connection

On January 23, 1998, researchers at the Harvard Medical School released a major study providing conclusive evidence that IGF-1 is a potent risk factor for prostate cancer. Should you be concerned? The only milk that would be safe to drink, although it has no health benefits even still, would be milk that is labeled "No rBGH and does not contain excess levels of IGF-1." American-made cheeses are contaminated with rBGH. Imported European cheeses are safe since Europe has banned rBGH.

Why Is American Milk Banned in Europe?

American dairy milk is genetically modified unless it is labeled "No rBGH."

Genetically engineered bovine growth hormone (rBGH) in milk increases cancer risks.

American dairy farmers inject dairy cows with rBGH to increase milk production. European nations and Canada have banned rBGH to protect citizens from 1GF-1 hazards. Monsanto Company, the manufacturer of rBGH, has influenced US product safety laws permitting the sale of unlabeled rBGH. Monsanto would lose billions of dollars if rBGH were banned in America.

Is there any milk not contaminated with rBGH and IGF-1? Yes, there is. Milk that is clearly labeled "NO rBGH" is free of rBGH and does not contain excess levels of IGF-1. American-made cheese is also contaminated with rBGH and excess levels of IGF-1 unless they are labeled "NO rBGH." Imported European cheeses are safe since Europe has banned rBGH. Remember, humans do not need cow's milk.

To research more information about America's dairy industry, there are many links (for example, www.milksucks.com). The FDA allows rBGH to endanger milk. To get the calcium and magnesium you need for your health today, you will need an organic calcium supplement. You can call our office to purchase our supplements that have stood the test of time for over fifty years. We can literally take the guesswork out of it for you. Milk for all mammal orphans is raw certified goat's milk. One way to find a source of the goat's milk is to go to your local chamber of commerce and ask who in your area buys goat feed.

2) TABLE SALT

The body needs sodium, but it must be in an organic form in order to be usable by the body. Table salt, sodium chloride, is an inorganic sodium compound formed by the union of sodium and chlorine that is extremely toxic to the body. This toxicity causes the body to retain fluid. Table salt contains aluminum, which can lead to senility and Alzheimer's. A healthy dosage for sodium is around one thousand milligrams. The USDA dietary guidelines will advise you to take more. A healthier choice would be sea salt used in the same proportion as regular salt. I also recommend potassium chloride instead of sodium chloride. You can sprinkle it on in the same way that you would regular sodium chloride.

3) SUGAR

The rise in sugar consumption parallels our increase in chronic degenerative diseases.

Everyone knows sugar is bad for you. But most have not given thought to how and why. The more sugar you eat, the more you will damage your health. The rise in sugar consumption parallels our increase in chronic degenerative diseases. Eating refined sugar throws the body into biochemical chaos. What does it do that is detrimental to your system? A mere teaspoon of refined sugar will cause the growth of several billion candida yeast in the blood stream. Imagine what it does when we eat more! Hardly anybody just consumes one teaspoon. Two teaspoons of sugar lowers the effectiveness of your immune system by 78 percent. So we can only guess what it would be if you had twelve teaspoons of sugar. So, somebody who feels a cold coming on and grabs the orange juice is actually sabotaging themselves without thinking about it. A better way to maintain your vitamin C levels is through eating fresh fruits and vegetables and taking a potent organic vitamin C supplement. I recommend and carry vitamin C that is the complete C complex as given to us in nature. It contains hesperidans, rutins, and bioflavonoids. God gave us a C complex which works much more effectively when it is taken as the complex all together. He also gave us a B complex, which must also be taken together as a complex. God gave us eight B vitamins that are to be taken together. You don't take a B12 or a B6 without also taking the whole B complex. The way our food is processed today, it's very difficult to get the nutrients we need. And that is where proper organic supplementation comes in.

Here are a few bits of information you might want to know about sugar:

Americans consume 150 pounds annually. That is thirty-three tablespoons a day, which is ninety-nine teaspoons daily. No wonder diabetes is one of the top killers in our nation. To envision that amount of sugar, try to visualize thirty 5-pound bags of sugar, and you will get an idea of how much you are eating a year. Schlotzsky's makes sandwiches which some people prefer to a hamburger because they think it is healthier. It has some vegetables in there, and it's on a whole grain bun, and it kind of looks like a meal, but it has a whopping twenty-eight grams of sugar! That contains about the same amount as a Snickers bar. Four grams of sugar equals one teaspoon (there are twenty-nine grams in four ounces of apple juice). That would be almost equivalent to a Snickers bar, which contains thirty grams of sugar or seven teaspoons. Just because it grew on a tree doesn't necessarily mean it won't have a huge impact on your insulin levels.

What about orange juice? That's a popular drink in the US. It's better, though, to eat an orange. To get four ounces of orange juice, you have to use four or five oranges. Often, at restaurants, they will serve you sixteen ounces of orange juice, so you are getting tons and tons of sugar. Yes, it is fruit sugar, but you don't benefit from taking it.

Refined, processed sugar is not a food at all. It is a toxic and addictive drug. Sugar is so changed and concentrated from its original plant form that it is actually a drug! Just ten teaspoons will immobilize the immune system by about 33 percent. Approximately thirty teaspoons of sugar will shut down the immune system for a whole day. Americans consume one cup of sugar daily.

Sugar is in practically all foods. And it does not come into our diets by the teaspoon of something, but through the trace amounts that are in our cereals, ketchup, baked goods, salad dressings, mayonnaise, cookies, and crackers. That's what causes the build-up in our bodies.

It has been said that sugar is the most dangerous food in the American diet. Dr. Ballantine, MD, a well-known doctor, has said, "For sugar to metabolize, it is so hard on the system that it draws nutrients from other parts of the body and leaves deficiencies for that food to digest. It puts a tremendous stress on the pancreas." Incidentally, cancer is a pancreatic enzyme deficiency. Remember, cancer cells love sugar. Cancer cells have six to ten times as many insulin receptor sites as healthy, well-differentiated cells. This allows cancer cells to feast on sugar. Remember, we all have cancer cells in our body. The health of our immune system is what determines whether or not those cancer cells will grow and multiply.

Summing up, sugar tastes so good, but it:
- Adds to risk of diabetes
- Increases body weight
- Is the cause of low blood sugar resulting in headaches, fatigue, light-headedness, and mood swings
- Creates a better environment to breed tumors
- Increases blood cholesterol
- Increases triglycerides
- Robs the body of necessary minerals
- Is like a parasite (it uses up vitamins)
- Promotes tooth decay
- Provides a lot of calories that are nutrient deficient
- Is usually combined with white flour, hydrogenated oils, and chemicals

- A major stress to the adrenal glands
- Feeds candida yeast

To break the sugar habit, try to eliminate all white sugar and flour for two weeks. Cravings will lessen. Get more bio-available vegetable protein, like our protein powders. Take a couple of organic multivitamins. Take four to six B complex and glucose regulating complex to control sugar cravings.

Dr. Yudkin, MD, has done a lot of research on sugar. He says that if everything were known that should be known about sugar, it would be automatically banned as a serious poison, and the FDA would not allow it in our foods. But the FDA is just too economically involved in it.

Instead of using white bleached sugar, you can put fructose in your sugar bowl, but only in moderation. Fructose is a simple sugar and is often referred to as fruit sugar. It is in a variety of foods. You can also use raw unfiltered honey or brown rice syrup. I think Stevia is a really important replacement for real sugar, especially for anyone who has candida, cancer, or any fungal problems. They should go to a form of sugar that does not affect that. Some Stevia can be a little bitter, but many of my patient/clients like the Sweet Leaf brand. Another sweetener you can try is Yacon root syrup. It is a great alternative to Stevia and any other sweeteners as well. Yacon is an Andean plant that is a relative of the sunflower. All of these alternatives are healthier choices for sugar—especially for those who are immune-system compromised. You will be the better off when you remove sugar from the diet.

It is no wonder that our children are so hyper and wired. Sugar can enlarge the kidneys and liver. Sugar robs the body of vitamin B and C and other essential nutrients like calcium. Eating sugar contributes to osteoporosis. Both white sugar and flour are among some of the leading causes of all disease. Why? Because they have been stripped of essential nutrients; they provide empty calories. White flour and white sugar are cheap fillers; consequently, they are in practically everything from fruit drinks to canned soups, mayonnaise, pickles, ketchup, soft drinks, cereals, and on and on, and we haven't even mentioned any desserts! There are nine teaspoons of sugar in a Coke.

What about some of the popular cereals? These are what the majority of American children eat for breakfast along with cow's milk. According to Sharon Broer's study on children's nutrition, Alpha-Bits cereal is 38 percent sugar, Frosted Flakes is 41 percent sugar, Life cereal is 16 percent sugar, Bran Flakes is 13 percent, and Fruit Loops is 48 percent sugar. Studies show that children who have an inadequate or sugary breakfast perform at lower levels in school. Our children today are being brainwashed by TV commercials. These are deceitful foods. God warned us to beware of deceitful foods. He says if you have an appetite for them put a knife to your throat! Proverbs 23:2 (this sounds serious!).

In 1973, Drs. Ringsdorf and Cheraskin noted a direct correlation in women and children between the frequency of infections (bacterial, urinary tract, yeast, and viral) and the amount of sugar consumed. Their findings, published in the *American Journal of Clinical Nutrition,* showed that the immune system actually shuts down when you give it sugar. They found that the equivalent of one piece of pie a la mode decreases your immune response by about 75 percent for four to six hours.

In conclusion, if you eat refined sugar morning, noon, and night, your body chemistry will be in chaos twenty-four hours a day. Cutting sugar out of your diet is a clear choice if you truly want to be healthy. The life of the flesh in is in the blood, and we want our blood to be more alkaline. Sugar is very acidic. The original health plan God gave us is alkaline.

4) REFINED FLOUR

At the turn of the century, the flourmill was invented, and heart disease and all degenerative diseases have increased steadily since.

Ninety-five percent of all the flour used in the US is refined white flour. Refined white flour and sugar are the main ingredients in most breakfast cereals and breakfast bars. When fed to laboratory animals, these food types will not support life, and the animals die. Whole unrefined grains will support life. A lot of people have switched from eating meat to eating more pasta, and they think they are doing their bodies a favor. But are they really? Most pasta is made from refined white flour. To make white flour, at least twenty-five nutrients are lost, while four are added back, and the flour is called "enriched." As someone has said, it should more accurately be called "impoverished." White flour does not produce healthy cells. There are pastas that are made from whole grains, and these are not perfect, but they are better than regular pasta. The very best choice would be to eat the fresh, unprocessed whole grains themselves. You can go to a health food store and buy many different organic whole grains. They can make a healthy addition to almost any diet. Once a grain has been ground into a fine powder, a lot of the nutrition has been lost. Refined flour has had all the good substances (bran and germ) removed during processing. Then it is bleached, sometimes with a bleaching agent similar to Clorox. Finally, some coal tar derived carcinogenic vitamins are added, and it is not a good food; in fact, it is hazardous to your health. Processed white flour and sugar will not support life. And yet, we eat them by the ton.

Think about what you are feeding your kids for lunch. And think of the refined foods that we give them for snacks. The refining process takes out all the nutrients. Breakfast foods are loaded with synthetic vitamins. Synthetic vitamins will never do you any good. If you are spending your money on synthetic vitamins, you truly are wasting your money. I cover this topic in greater detail in another chapter.

Our breakfast foods and many other grains are steamed and rolled and puffed, and then they are filled with sugary things. White flour is a poison. Wheat builds flab; rye builds muscle. There are other grains that are healthier and protect the cells from cancer. Wheat, corn, and milk are highly allergic foods. All the corn in our nation is GMO. I do not recommend eating any corn at all at this point.

A good bread should only have five or six ingredients, and that is it. We are tricked by the food industry, as they put about ninety chemicals in the breads and flours. And then they call it enriched. That's like a robber coming up to me and grabbing my purse and when I scream and cry and holler, he comes back and gives me a Kleenex or comb out of my purse.

A lot of my clients like the Ezekiel 4:9 bread, which is found in the refrigerated or frozen food section of the grocery store. It is refrigerated because it is a live food. It is a Bible food. Many will make their delicious protein smoothie with the protein powders we carry, and then they will make a slice or two of Ezekiel's toast with the cinnamon raisin recipe of Ezekiel's bread. It is delicious with a little bit of regular unsalted butter spread on top. Whole grain and bread mixes made by Arrowhead Mills are also a healthy choice.

5) ALUMINIUM CANS

Foods in an aluminum can are a "dead food." They have nothing that can promote health or life. They may be able to keep one alive, but they do not promote health. I keep some canned foods in case we have a major crisis. On the side of the can it may list vitamins, but they are synthetic. The human body knows the difference. Canned food contributes to Alzheimer's among other conditions; there is no life in a canned food. Aren't we supposed to be eating to promote health and vitality?

6) ARTIFICIAL SWEETENERS

Which do you like—the pink, the blue, or the yellow? No, I am not talking about newborn colors, but about artificial sweeteners. I do not allow them in my house. So what does that tell you? Artificial sweeteners are a neurotoxin to the brain. The CDC has had more complaints connected to artificial sweeteners than any other product on the market. Artificial sweeteners can cause headaches, migraines, memory lapses, brain tumors, aneurisms, seizures, and obesity. And it is happening every day. Seventy percent of Americans are overweight and consume a lot of diet sodas. Artificial sweeteners keep you fat, and the soft drinks give you soft bones. Is that what you really want?

7) HOT DOGS AND ALL PROCESSED LUNCH MEATS WITH NITRATES AND NITRITES

You have a 6,700 percent greater chance of getting pancreatic and stomach cancer when you eat cold cuts. Children who eat hot dogs increase their risk of cancer greatly.

We have already discussed how detrimental to our health eating any pork products is . . . this is just a reminder to not eat cold cuts and hot dogs.

CHAPTER 7

Clarification of New Testament Scriptures

A Lot of Confusion

We have been misled in the body of Christ. In this chapter we will clarify those stumbling block Scriptures.

Did you know there are six hundred Scriptures in the Bible pertaining to health: foods to eat for health, foods that will kill if we eat them, and also on how to live long and well on the earth?

I had someone come up to me after a seminar at a church in Dallas who said, "I had no idea that the Bible had anything to say about my grocery list!" As we have heard for so long, "My people (not somebody else's people) are perishing for lack of knowledge" (Hosea 4:6).

Let's note the very last chapter in the Bible. In Revelation 22:2, the apostle John addresses the healing of leaves for the nations and offers "the fruit of the month" for food and the leaves of the tree for the healing of the nations. From the first chapter to the last and in every chapter in between, God is telling us how to live, thrive, and be successful—body, soul, and spirit—in life. And remember *Father Knows Best?* He really does! We want our children to believe that about our instructions, and He wants us to believe that about His instructions. But Hosea says we are lacking in that knowledge, and so, we suffer.

How Are the Old Testament and the Law Related to the New Testament and Today's Believer?

What position did Jesus, the apostles, and the early church take on this question? It is very important that we rightly settle this in our minds in order to keep ourselves from error, frustration, and even serious trouble and heartache. This needs to move from being an opinion to being a heartfelt conviction. The Bible does not contradict itself; Jesus is the same yesterday, today, and forever. God's laws are very consistent throughout the Old Testament and the New Testament that it may go well with us. He has not changed them. His laws are just as relevant for His children today. For example, Genesis 8:22 states that as long as the earth remains, there is seed time, and then there is harvest. These are laws for while we are on the earth.

The Bible is a two-edged sword; both the Old and the New Testaments are essential to our lives. The Old Testament is God's truth enfolded; in the New, it is unfolded to the nations. In the Old Testament, events are predicted; in the New, they are (or ultimately will be) fulfilled. In the Old, the Messiah is concealed; in the New, He is revealed. The Old is the root; the New is the branch. The Old is the bud; the New is the flower. The New Testament is impossible without the Old, like leaves and fruit without the branch and tree. One is the counterpart of the other; both are incomplete without the other.

Matthew

What did Jesus think about the law? Some people say the law has passed away. But what does Jesus say?

In Matthew 5:17–19 Jesus says, "Do not think I have come to abolish the Law or the Prophets; I have not come to abolish them but to fulfill them." Instead of minimizing the law, Jesus actually magnified it as revealed in this passage. He fulfilled the law perfectly, or He could not have been the transgressor's substitute and sin offering (Isaiah 53).

And again, Jesus said about the law, "Do not think I have come to abolish the Law or the Prophets; I have not come to abolish them but to fulfill them. For assuredly I say to you, till heaven and earth pass away, one jot or one tittle will by no means pass from the law till all is fulfilled." To destroy means to abolish or rob of its power, but Jesus said these laws are with us until the end of the age for our good while we are on the earth. Can you imagine someone jumping off a 40-story high building and saying all the way down, "I'm free of the law!"? When they splatter on the ground, if they are in Jesus Christ, they are going to heaven, but the law of gravity is still in effect, and all the laws of God are that way as well. I can know Jesus but not obey the laws of God and it will still affect me in my life and body while on this earth. This has everything to do with being blessed while on the earth and has nothing to do with a requirement for salvation or getting into heaven. Our salvation comes through believing in Jesus Christ by faith and that alone.

What Was Jesus' Attitude Toward God's Holy Dietary Law?

First, we know He observed the law, or He could not have been the world's redeemer. He had to fulfill all the divine requirements of the law completely in order to be the perfect sacrifice, without the least condemnation, sin, or guilt. There is never a record where He ate anything unclean or violated the healthful nutritional laws of God; if He had, He could not have faced the throng with the query, "Which of you convicts me of transgression?"

In three of the gospels, we have the story of Jesus crossing the Sea of Galilee and coming to the country of the Gadarenes. As He came ashore, a man met Him who was possessed by demons. He could not be chained or tamed by any man, and he was naked and dwelt among the tombs. Jesus commanded these unclean spirits to come out of the man, and He sent them into a herd of swine feeding nearby. The herd immediately ran violently down a steep place into the sea and perished. Mark tells us there were about two thousand hogs that choked in the sea.

What Was the Apostle Paul's and King David's Opinion about the Law?

Let's look at Romans 8:4: "That the righteousness of the law might be fulfilled in us, who walk not after the flesh but after the spirit."

Romans 7:12, 14 tells us that the law is holy, just, good, and spiritual. It is for our benefit. Paul writes (as did King David), "I delight in the law of God; I love the law."

Peter's Vision

This passage has misled Christians and kept them sick for a long time.

Have you heard about Peter's vision? Acts 10: 9–28 has always been a stumbling block passage with regard to this subject. Consider verse 9: "The next day, as they went on their journey and drew near the city, Peter went up on the housetop to pray, about the sixth hour. Then he became very hungry and wanted to eat: but while they made ready, he fell into a trance. Heaven opened and an object like a great sheet bound at the four corners descended to him and let down to the earth. In it were all kinds of four-footed animals of the earth, wild beasts, creeping things, and birds of the air. And a voice came to him, 'Rise, kill, and eat.' Peter answered, 'Not so, Lord, for I have never eaten anything unclean.'" Because Peter was a Jew, he knew it did not mean that he could eat unclean animals.

So, What Was the Meaning of the Vision?

As you read on down in the chapter, verse 28 states that God has shown Peter the meaning of the vision, *which was not to call any man unclean*; it had nothing to do with dietary laws. While Peter is wondering about the meaning of the vision, we've made up our minds that we can eat anything we want as long as we pray over it with the mindset that we are not under the law. But in verse 28, Peter speaks the meaning of the vision: to not call any *man unclean. The Lord is dealing with people in the vision—not pigs!*

This chapter is about God using Peter, a Jew, to go to the home of Cornelius, a gentile, and take the gospel. It has nothing to do with dietary suggestions. God is calling him as a leader of the early church out of being prejudiced against gentiles. The unclean animals are representative of the nations to which God is sending the gospel. The animals were merely figures and types. For example:

America—The Eagle (Unclean Animal)
Russia—The Bear (Unclean Animal)
England—The Lion (Unclean Animal)

We need to learn to not take Scriptures out of context. God is preparing Peter, a Jew, to affirm taking the gospel to the gentile nations with love and acceptance, not prejudice. God did not change the gastric juices of our bodies nor of the unclean beasts. He did not perform a biological miracle in these unclean animals so that we could eat them and not suffer. The unclean animals in the air, land, and waters are scavengers. They were put here with a purpose—to clean up the planet of all the dead, diseased animals in the air, land, and waters. They were not created for us to eat; however, had He not created the garbage collectors, disease would proliferate and mankind would die off.

Whether you look at it from a biochemical point of view or a biophysical one, when we eat any of the unclean meat, it causes the levels of blood ureas to rise too quickly. It's interesting that the foods God told us we could eat do not have this adverse effect in the body.

So, What Happens When You Eat the Unclean Animals?

As previously mentioned, you have an almost immediate rise in blood ureas, which means that the food is being digested too quickly and the body cannot assimilate it. It causes the blood protein to digest too fast; it increases the viscosity of the blood and raises blood pressure. It also increases heart rate and aging. This is one of the reasons why so many believers are ill.

Merely praying over your food is not working. I actually heard about an overweight woman who went to a restaurant and ordered the most fattening food on the menu plus a dessert. As they set her food before her, she bowed her head and prayed and asked God to bless her meal and take away the calories. That theology is not working. In fact, it is sheer witchcraft, because God created our bodies and He created the system that does work. It is called Exodus 15:26: "If you will listen to me and obey me, and do what I say, I will be your health, for I am the God that heals you." And then He immediately begins to bless their food and water. God cannot be mocked. Whatsoever we sow, we do reap, and that is a law that is with us until the end of the age. It doesn't matter whether you believe it or not. It doesn't matter whether you like it or not!

Another Scripture that has been fearfully misinterpreted by certain Bible readers is in 1 Timothy. Paul writes to young Timothy: "Now the spirit speaks expressly that in the latter times, some shall depart from the faith, giving heed to seducing spirits, and doctrines of devils; speaking lies in hypocrisy; having their conscience seared with a hot iron, forbidding to marry, and commanding to abstain from meats, which God has created to be received with thanksgiving of them which believe and know the truth. For every creature of God is good, and nothing is to be refused, if it is received with thanksgiving. For it is sanctified by the word of God and prayer" (1 Timothy 4:1-5).

By carefully considering the context of these words, we find nothing out of harmony with the rest of the Scriptures. Apparently, some specific end-time group is described that forbids marriage, is full of hypocrisy, and is demon-controlled. In addition, this group commands its followers to abstain from obviously clean food, which God has created to be received with thanksgiving of them which believe and know the actual truth.

My purpose here is not to dwell on the identity of these evil perverters of the gospel, but to dispel the idea that merely praying over food can make it good to eat. Paul affirms that any created thing in the food line or department is acceptable as long as it meets two tests:

1) It must be approved (or sanctified) by the Bible.

2) It should be prayed over with thanksgiving.

Please take note that both of these requirements must be met in order for the food to be suitable for the Christian diet. Incidentally, the word "meats" in the original language is not limited to flesh foods. The Greek word *broma* simply means "food."

Do these verses suggest that moles, bats, and rattlesnakes may be sanctified for food by simply praying over them? Quite the opposite! Nothing is made suitable unless it has passed the first test of being approved by the Word of God. If the Bible says it is clean, then and only then can prayers of thanksgiving be assured the seal of God's acceptance.

I encourage you to read it in its entirety. But I want to call your attention to the word "foods" there. In an exhaustive concordance, the word "foods" refers back to Leviticus where the clean and unclean foods are delineated. The Judaizers were saying that beef was unclean. God said that beef is clean; of course, today it is filled with hormones and antibiotics. But the way beef is created by God, it is a clean animal and can be eaten. However, beef was only to be eaten once in a while for celebrations. You'll note that for their celebrations, it was "let's kill the fatted calf," not the fatted pig! And biblically, beef was only eaten for celebrations. Their staple was Genesis 1:29 and 30: fresh fruits, vegetables, whole grains, raw nuts, and raw seeds.

When 1 Timothy was written, all they had was the Torah, the first five books of the Bible. Where in the first five books of the Bible does it say you can eat whatever you want and it will be sanctified by the Word of God?

1 Peter 1:16: "Be holy as I am holy." If you look at the concordance, it refers back to Leviticus 11:44, 45—clean and unclean foods.

1 Peter 2:9: "We have been set apart. We are a chosen people, a royal priesthood, a holy nation, a people belonging to God, to declare the praises of Him who called you out of darkness into His wonderful light. We have been set apart as was Daniel from the world and its delicacies."

1 John 2:3–6: "He, who abides in Him, ought also to walk as He walked. He is our example in everything." Did Jesus eat any unclean food? If He had, He would not have been able to be the perfect sacrifice and die for us. Did the apostles and the disciples eat any unclean

meat? I think they knew better. And our anatomy is the same as theirs.

2 Corinthians 6:17: "Come out from among them and be ye separate and touch not the unclean thing." This passage in the New Testament refers back to Isaiah 52:11, which refers back to the commandments of God and clean and unclean. I was raised in a strong Christian home and always taught that this passage means "Don't drink, don't play cards, don't touch a boy, and don't go to movies!" But the actual meaning is, "Don't eat pork chops, ham, shrimp, and devil's food chocolate cake!" Something altogether different. We have been set apart in every way.

Proverbs 23:2: "If you are a man given to appetite, put a knife to your throat." God is serious about bringing our body into subjection.

In 1 Corinthians 9:27, Paul says, "I bring my body in subjection, lest I be considered a counterfeit." And sometimes our taste buds are the last thing to come under the control and be yielded to the Holy Spirit.

In Philippians 3:19, Paul warns about our appetite or our bellies being our god. Does your appetite control you? If so, "God says our mind is then set on the flesh and earthly things and ends in destruction."

Can God revitalize your body? Can He change you? If you have overcome the addiction of smoking, God did a miracle for you. And He can revitalize your taste buds. There is no condemnation here, but as a Christian family, we want to be informed on how to live out our number of days, not three score and ten but over one hundred years in health and enjoying life. It is God's heart and desire for His children.

CHAPTER 8

What About Supplements?

Are All Vitamins Created Equal?

Are Supplements an Option?

Given the fact we aren't getting the nutrients we need in our foods alone and that the soil is depleted, people often ask me about vitamin and mineral supplementation. Given the fact that our supply of nutrients is down and our need is up, I believe supplements are an essential part of virtually everyone's eating plan for health. Given the fact we don't eat enough raw fresh fruits and vegetables (and the ones we do eat, many times we are not digesting well), it is important that we supplement for prevention and healing.

Real food (especially raw fresh fruits and vegetables) is always the best, but given the poor quality of our so-called food today, I take daily selective supplements and recommend them to my clients. I am extremely selective in the quality and efficacy of what I offer my clients. Supplements are no panacea, as many supplements do not assimilate. Because competition in the vitamin industry is based on price, most manufacturers cut corners and aim at lowering the cost of their product rather than increasing its safety and efficacy. Very few suppliers have any idea of the technology required to produce a supplement that conforms to good science and efficacy (the ability to produce a desired result). In fact, 80 percent of people who take supplements don't even notice any difference when they take them. Why is that? Because most supplements contain only a small portion of the active ingredient. Clients come into my office with bags of "supplements" they have spent many dollars on, and they come to see me because they are not well. I then ask them what each one is for, and they don't even know. There are only a few brands of supplements that I can recommend.

This chapter is to help answer every question you ever wanted to ask about supplements. Before we begin, please note that the supplements and guidelines I recommend are based solely on the supplements that we have researched. In a health food store, there are literally hundreds of bottles with labels claiming wonderful benefits, but *few have been clinically tested, so it's guesswork. I learned this the hard way.* The FDA does not require testing. More and more research is revealing that septic tanks are clogged with undigested vitamin pills. One client (who told me she had previously been on a lot of different vitamin pills) said the plumber told her they found the cause of her blocked-up septic tank. They proceeded to show her hundreds of undigested one-a-day vitamins; some of them still had their brand names readable!

One interesting case study was published by the *Annals of Pharmacotherapy* in 1992, (Issue 26), it featured a patient complaining of abdominal discomfort, which was caused by forty to fifty intact pills forming a large single mass in her colon. The mass was attributed to vitamin supplements she had purchased at a health food store.

It seems everywhere we turn, we see advertisements for all sorts of vitamins. Are they really necessary? And how do we know which ones really work?

Your body contains trillions of cells. And we make about sixty million new cells every minute of every day. We replace most of the cells in our body every year. Trillions of new cells are created every day. Each cell is like a high-performance engine. It needs high quality raw materials (nutrients) to function properly. The quantity and quality of nutrients you ingest affects every system in your body: cardiovascular, digestive, muscular, skeletal, lymphatic, endocrine, reproductive, urinary, and even your nervous system. In other words, how you look, feel, and perform is directly affected by your daily nutrient intake.

Your Body Can't Manufacture All the Nutrients It Needs on Its Own Alone

Scientists define a vitamin as a compound essential for life. And since your body cannot manufacture most of these vitamins on its own, they can only come from the food you eat and the supplements you take every day. Over the long term, proper nutrition impacts every aspect of your health—from its ability to maintain health to its role in preventing nutrition-related diseases such as heart disease and diabetes. If you are not on a good, healthy nutritional plan, wouldn't it be a good idea to start now?

We simply can't get what we need in our foods alone in today's world. Even if you had an organic garden out your back door, you still need to selectively supplement. And here are some of the reasons why. In America, we have not been obedient to God's principles for health. We haven't rested our soil since the thirties. Most of us hear admonishments to eat more fresh fruits and vegetables for better nutrition, but where do the fresh fruits and vegetables get their nutrients? From the soil, of course. And since we have not rested our soil for over eighty years, our soil is depleted. And then, God told us to not mingle the seed. The seed in our nation is hybrid seed, which produces an inferior crop. And then you have atomic hydrogen bomb stuff coming out of the air. Early harvesting and the long transporting of produce make it necessary to supplement. Another noteworthy point is that we are not merely trying to prevent scurvy (vitamin C deficiency) or rickets (vitamin D deficiency); we need to be supplementing to prevent cancer, heart disease, diabetes, arthritis and osteoporosis. *These are our top killers today.*

God gave us food; He never intended that we would have to take food supplements, but man has so polluted God's food that in order to prevent getting cancer and getting ill, we have to selectively supplement. *It's nice to know we have a solution.*

Our food is not what it used to be. As someone has said, in today's world, we have fast food, frozen food, processed food, and then we have live, healthy food. In other words, there is devil's food and there is angel's food. We can choose. Do you want to be like the devil or one of God's agents?

If the cells of the body are made up of organic vitamins, minerals, and amino acids, where are we getting those nutrients from today's food choices? Most of the food we eat hardly resembles real food. It has been washed, cut, sliced, mashed, mangled, loaded with additives, waxed, and then popped into a microwave, which destroys all the life. Any animal protein in that microwaved food becomes carcinogenic (cancer forming), by the way.

According to research, only about 3 percent of the population even begins to eat a balanced meal, according to the food guide pyramid guidelines. Only 9 percent of adults consume five fresh fruits and vegetables daily. Forty-five percent eat no fruit or fruit juice; 48 percent eat no vegetables or only one serving (and that included French fries). If eating a diet of fresh plant foods is what we *should* be doing, let's have a fresh look at what we are *actually* doing. According to the US Bureau of Labor statistics, the average US household now spends $4,399 per year on groceries. Out of more than $4,000 spent on food, only $132 per year is spent on fresh produce. Do we need to look any further as to why there is so much chronic disease, and why we must be selective in our supplementation? We carry one supplement that has the seed benefit of thousands of fresh fruits and vegetables in just one capsule.

If you didn't see it before, are you now beginning to understand why we need to supplement with the proper food supplements (not just any) for better health? It is very difficult for most to get what they need in their food alone. And most are not.

The average person eats one serving daily of fruit and 1.8 servings of vegetables—only 0.7 if you exclude fried potatoes and lettuce and tomatoes as a garnish to fast food. To put things in better perspective, consider what happens nutritionally in America on an average day:

- 16,300,000 eat at McDonald's.
- 1,700,000 children eat at a hamburger chain.
- 2,740,000 Dunkin' donuts are eaten.
- Americans eat 24,700,000 hot dogs.
- Americans spend $10,411,000 on potato chips.

We've had a 2,000 percent increase in fast food sales over the past thirty years.

One-third of our total calories comes from fast food, which is lacking in good nutrition. Not only does high fat, high carbohydrate fast food deliver a lot of calories, but the latest research shows that it also may result in acute inflammation. And consuming these high fat, high calorie fast food meals regularly may lead to chronic inflammation, which may put you at risk for many diseases, including heart disease, diabetes, arthritis, certain cancers, and Alzheimer's disease.

Eating Right Isn't As Easy As It Seems . . . But It Is Possible

Ninety-eight percent of Americans do not eat the recommended seven to nine servings of fruits and vegetables each day. What might surprise you even more is that even when you try to do the right thing, the nutritional value of our produce isn't what it used to be. Remember the old adage, "an apple a day keeps the doctor away"? Today it is twenty-six apples a day because of the decline in nutritional value in the produce. In fact, a 2004 study of forty-three crops showed a decline in the nutrient content of up to 38 percent over the past fifty years. Ninety percent of Americans fall short in getting essential nutrients in their diets.

Countless Studies Can't All Be Wrong

Many of the world's leading experts in medicine, biochemistry, and nutrition believe nutritional supplementation positively affects overall health. Doctors and researchers from Harvard, Stanford, Yale, the American Heart Association, and the American Cancer Society can't all be wrong. If you want to improve your health, be sure to get some of the most important nutrients your body and your brain need to function optimally: a multivitamin, vitamin D3, calcium, B vitamins, vitamin C, Omega-3 fatty acids, antioxidants, and probiotics.

How many of us consume thirty-five grams of soluble fiber a day? The lack of fiber in our diet can be deadly. Without it, cancer of both the colon and bowel are more likely, as well as constipation, hemorrhoids, diverticulosis, varicose veins, heart disease, appendicitis, gall bladder disease, and hiatal hernia, just to name a few.

Americans eat too much fat and sugar. When you look at what children are eating on Saturday mornings, they are consuming what is being advertised on television: fats, oils, and sweets—no fresh fruit or vegetables are being advertised. Is it any wonder that the number one cause of death in children under the age of thirteen is cancer, next to accidents?

If you can't get these nutrients in your diet, if you won't get them in your diet, if you don't like broccoli, then take supplements to make up the difference. Food supplements are no substitute, however, for a poor diet. Supplements are only part of the solution, but they *are a very important one.* Today we are not merely trying to prevent scurvy (vitamin C deficiency) or beriberi (B1 deficiency); we need to prevent cancer, heart disease, arthritis, and diabetes, too. **The guidelines on vitamin bottles are put there by the FDA and are minimal RDI to prevent rickets, scurvy, or beriberi.** They do not have the therapeutic dosages for food supplements to prevent all of the top killers. Who wants minimal health? I believe most of us would prefer optimal health!

Is There Any Proof That Taking Vitamins Will Work?

Often, I hear from my patient/clients that their doctors have told them there is nothing they could have done to prevent or to heal their conditions. They also are being told that the food they eat or do not eat has no bearing on or correlation to their disease. This has been the official position of orthodox medicine—that there is no association whatsoever between nutrition and one's health. In fact, the Arthritis Foundation and most doctors, in general, will say that there is nothing in the diet that will affect (either improve or cause) arthritic flare-ups or cancer or any disease. For the record, any doctor or person who makes a statement like that has not done his professional homework.

When I counsel someone, I want them to know exactly what foods will heal them, what foods are killing them, what each needed supplement's purpose is, and how you should take each supplement. When my clients walk out of my office or hang up the phone from a phone consultation, they know exactly how to take charge of their condition to get well and healthy based on my years of working with people successfully with that respective condition. If you are buying supplements, I encourage you to make sure the person you are paying for your vitamins has helped many people get well from whatever issues are concerning you. **Whomever you are buying your supplements from should also be helping you with your quality of health, life, and longevity.** They should be helping you avoid getting our top killers like cancer through advising you on proper supplementation, foods you should eat and what foods you need to avoid.

I never carried products in my nutritional practice until I, along with 1,500 other people, was poisoned on a product from a health food store. Most of those people died. Had I not had the knowledge of how to heal the body of almost any disease, I would have died, too. The poisoning came from a contaminated batch out of Japan. I learned the hard way that the FDA does not require any of those labels and brands at health food stores or vitamin shops to be clinically tested for purity, safety, and efficacy, *so they are not.*

When you are shopping at the health food store or Costco or the drug store, you are spending your hard-earned money, but you are guessing. I learned the hard way that *guessing can be very dangerous.* It is not necessary to guess when there are products available that are pure and are clinically tested to deliver the goods of health, vitality, and efficacy and promote long life on the cellular level.

Since that event, God has led me to supplements I can trust, and they have given me back my life after nearly dying from the poisoning. I now write out people's nutritional plans, and they have the option of getting their supplements from me or going to the health food store and buying them. If they go to the health food store, they are guessing, *but that is their choice.* We now offer a healthier option. Most want to take advantage of what I carry because they have been confused on this subject. The companies I now recommend and offer in my practice have set the standards in the world of supplements for over fifty years.

Sixty percent of Americans are taking some form of supplements. **However, only about 5 percent of Americans are in the range of happiness and feeling well.** One-third of the 60 percent are consuming various synthetic vitamins like Centrum, Theragram M, and Flintstone vitamins which say "Keep out of the reach of children" because they are toxic. Even our adult vitamins do not have this label on them. What does that tell you? They are just good food. And that is what our bodies need.

So, What Kind of Vitamins Do You Take?

Would they be classified as a food or a drug?

Have they been clinically tested for purity, efficacy, and safety? Or are you just grabbing a bottle of vitamins while you are shopping and assuming they will work for you?

Would the FDA classify them as a food or a drug? If you are spending money on supplements, these are important questions to have answered.

Is there a difference between synthetic and organic? Yes, there is. All vitamins are not created equal. Sixty percent of Americans are taking supplements on a regular basis; 70 percent take them most of the time. But are you well? People are paying a lot of money for supplements; yet many may be wasting their money. Are they really getting the results they want and deserve? Or are you moving at a fast pace on the slippery slope along with most Americans?

A truly natural supplement is one that is a concentrated food source. When you look at the label, you should recognize food sources, for example, fish oil, alfalfa, brewer's yeast, wheat germ oil, lecithin, and desiccated liver.

However, many of the supplements today are derived from a synthetic source; that is, a laboratory product whose molecular structure is similar to the supplement being copied. Synthetic supplements are used because of the cost or availability of a natural commercial source. Synthetic vitamins are processed with coal tar and high heat which kills the life and destroys the enzymes.

Let's take vitamin E, for example: the natural one is from soy (a real food source); the synthetic one is from petroleum. The natural source is about five times more potent than the synthetic source, so you are not getting your money's worth if you are buying synthetic vitamin E. The drug store, the grocery store; stores like Costco, Walmart, and some vitamin shops; even some health food stores and Target would carry synthetic. And not only synthetic but supplements that are not clinically tested for purity, safety, and efficacy. For a label to say "100 percent natural," it only has to contain 10 percent of the actual substance.

Let's look at vitamin C. Studies show that the correct amount of a quality vitamin C product will reduce the risk of cataracts by 77-83% and in one UCLA study, it helped men live an additional six years. But to get that amount of vitamin E and C in your food, you'd have to eat six oranges a day and a couple of jars of wheat germ to get that much nutrient. The value here is that the vitamin pills are a wonderful supplement to a very good diet, and they'll add these benefits over and above what you can consume. Just think of the calories you can spare by supplementing.

Guidelines for Choosing Vitamins

There are all kinds of supplements on the market; there are hundreds of companies that are willing to take your money and sell you something. Many have jumped on the bandwagon and are selling all sorts of so-called health products. Most of these have not been clinically tested for purity, safety, and efficacy. The FDA does not require companies and brands at health food stores or anywhere where supplements are sold to be clinically tested, so they are not.

Some might find it a bit confusing when roaming a health food store. There might be dozens of B6 alone, and they may be in dozens of strengths. This can be overwhelming.

Basically there are three types of processing for the vitamins in our nation:

1) Test tube or synthetic vitamins: these are the ones I call artificial. These are the ones that you see most commonly at grocery stores, vitamin or herb shops, and some health food stores. These are the ones that are heavily advertised on television, and in magazines.

Without listing some of the most popular vitamin labels, most have the label "Keep out of the reach of children." Even the number one chewable children's vitamin on the market says "Keep out of the reach of children" on them. That is because they are toxic. And it is worth repeating that our adult supplements do not say "Keep out of the reach of children" on them. Why? Because they are just good unadulterated food. And you know the FDA would require it to be there if our supplements were toxic in any way. The question about the synthetic vitamins is, are they clinically tested to do what they are supposed to do and what you are looking for in benefiting your health? The answer is most likely that they are not. Some companies, if you inquire, may say the clinical studies are pending, but it is likely they do not have any research of their own. This has been our experience through the years as we have written to different companies for the clinical research and typically, hear nothing back. Personally, *I don't want to be guessing while their studies are pending!*

Synthetic vitamins made from a test tube are made from coal tar. They don't deliver the goods when it comes to your health. They are made from coal tar derivatives. That putrid smell you get when you open up a bottle of synthetics is the coal tar. It's the petroleum derivatives. Coal tar is that black sludge in the bottom of the barrel after they've made gasoline out of crude oil. If you are not quite convinced, just stick them in the oven at about 250 degrees for about three minutes. That black coal tar comes boiling up out of the tablet. You can try this at home. One of the problems is that people have a lot of side effects just from the coal tar. When you spend money on a supplement, don't you want benefits, not toxic side effects?

NYU did an experiment on all their athletes to see if taking synthetic vitamins improved their athletic performance. They split their athletic teams in half. Half took them and half did not to see if there was a difference, and there was. There was a marked difference. The people who took the synthetic vitamins did significantly worse than those who took nothing at all.

It's business people or pharmaceutical companies that design the contents of these synthetic vitamins, which are high in concentration. Those that are expensive and more important are low or absent. Two vitamins that are very expensive to synthesize and are very important are biotin and folic acid, both B vitamins. And are all the vitamins and percentages recommended by the FDA actually present?

Also, is it balanced? All vitamins have been given a percent of RDI (recommended dietary intake), and all the percentages are the same, no matter what they are. Keep in mind there are three vitamins—thiamine, riboflavin, and niacin—that are extremely cheap to manufacture. When you see flour, pasta, or bread labeled "enriched," it simply means that all the vitamins and minerals have been removed. They take out twenty-three and then put back three. That's robbery!

Without my mentioning it, you probably know what the number one vitamin supplement sold in our country is. But is it complete? It has no folic acid and no biotin (both very important), so it's incomplete. Look at the list for recommended daily allowance, and it has anywhere from zero all the way up to the three cheapies that go 500 percent, 588 percent, and 687 percent of the RDA in a single tablet. So what you have in these is a lot of the cheap and none of the expensive. The high percentages of the cheap can make it misleading.

Let's look at the ingredients by volume. The number one ingredient by volume is SUGAR. There is absolutely no value in having sugar in a vitamin tablet. I question the motivation of anyone who would put sugar in a vitamin supplement. And then, on down the line, is sodium ascorbate, calcium carbonate (a filler). Ascorbate is synthetic vitamin C. Number five on the list is talc, and talc is glass; talcum powder is ground glass. Now, they don't have an RDA in the human body for silicon—it's a binder and used to keep the pill from falling apart. The next in line is lactose: that is sugar, which is used as a filler. Cellulose is a filler; gelatin is a filler; acacia, which is a natural form of gum, is a filler; and starch is a filler. So how much actual vitamin or mineral is in here? It contains mostly fillers that are cheap to manufacture. Now, there is also shellac, which keeps the supplement from dissolving too quickly. Again, there's not an RDA for shellac in the human body. On down the list are more fillers and waxes and binders, so it's no wonder you get stomach aches when you take vitamins like these.

The chemical or imitation vitamin is the end product of a chemist's test tube. Chemical or synthetic vitamins are made from coal tar derivatives and are inorganic. And the body does know the difference. Biochemists as well as medical scientists proved long ago that synthetic vitamins cannot become a part of human tissue as they are inorganic, and the body will reject them. It is true that a chemical vitamin may stimulate or nudge a sick or lazy cell, but it will not feed and nourish it. Chemical vitamins are the cheapest, but they're also the least effective. We also know that coal tar derivatives can create cancer in laboratory animals.

To further illustrate this point, a group of British scientists in conjunction with Jacques Cousteau tried to simulate sea water. Once they had done this, they took fish and introduced them to an aquarium with the simulated seawater in a laboratory environment. Not surprisingly, the fish could not live. The scientists kept trying to make it perfect, but the fish kept dying in the synthetic seawater. Finally, they added two tablespoons of natural seawater to the aquarium to give life to these fish. There is something life-giving in natural seawater that is not in synthetic seawater that is so minute that the scientists could not even identify it or see it under a microscope, so they couldn't synthesize it.

The synthetic or plastic vitamins are classified as a drug by the FDA.

2) The second type of vitamins are the crystalline or organic extract

variety, and ***these are the ones in the health food stores.*** To make natural vitamin C by the extract method, you take an orange, grind it up into a slimy pulp, and mix it with acetone. After it's heated, the vapor that comes off it condenses, and you get this white crystalline powder at the bottom. You have extracted, roughly speaking, the vitamin C. What you may not realize is that in nature and in foods, there is a whole group of compounds, called bioflavonoids. There are over two hundred bioflavonoids that boost vitamin C. When you get the whole complex, the benefit is much greater than if you take just an extracted vitamin C.

Again, these vitamins are made by business people, and many times, they are neither balanced nor scientifically sound. Many times, the FDA only requires 10 percent of the tablet content to come from a natural source to be labeled natural. The rest can be synthetic. It can even have the cold tar in it and still be labeled as natural as long as 10 percent comes from a natural source.

The crystalline (powdered) or altered vitamin comes from natural sources, but has been isolated by heating to temperatures beyond 160 degrees. This destroys much of the natural enzymes that occur in nature. When a vitamin has been concentrated down to provide two hundred to five hundred or more milligrams per tablet, heat must be applied, and the entire molecular balance created by nature is completely destroyed. Also, to get such concentration in tablet form, many of the nutrients that occur naturally are removed, if not destroyed. Here again is man tampering with nature to produce a cheaper product—one that can remain on a shelf for indefinite periods of time without spoiling. This fact in itself should tell us something. The crystalline or isolates are classified as a drug by the FDA.

And then there is a third kind of processing. This is what we believe in, recommend, and offer. The FDA classifies these as a food . . . they do not even say "keep out of the reach of children" on them.

3) A third kind of supplement is the natural, unaltered, or food concentrate kind. This type takes the vitamin and mineral-rich food, for example, Brewer's yeast and alfalfa leaves, and concentrates it into

tablet form. The fiber and water are removed and within that tablet form is everything that was in the food to begin with. The balance that exists in nature exists in the tablet, and there are very few companies I know of that actually do this. The supplements we order do and have stood the test of time for over fifty years.

These supplements are just plain unadulterated concentrated food, in complete balance with nature. Nothing has been removed except the water and any cellulose fiber. The natural materials have not been exposed to temperatures beyond 100 degrees, thereby preserving the natural balance and enzymes that occur in nature. They are formulated by what is known as the "cold process." These supplements contain no preservatives, additives, chemicals, or fillers. Because the materials used are natural foods, the quality control must be extremely rigid, so this is a more expensive process. Organic materials vary and can spoil. The shelf life of our supplements are said to be around six months.

Deborah Norville, of NBC's *Today Show*, once interviewed Bonnie Liebman, nutrition director of the Center for Science in the Public Interest. Ms. Liebman cautioned that the lack of standards for testing nutritional supplements means that many manufacturers may not accurately test for disintegration time to ensure their products actually provide the nutrients claimed on their labels. She did an experiment on several types of supplements. Of the numerous multivitamin and multi-mineral supplements tested, some took over an hour or more to dissolve, while our multivitamin took only seventeen minutes to break down. The testing was done by Howard University's School of Pharmacy, using testing standards which were based on governmentally mandated tests for pharmaceuticals.

The FDA classifies these vitamins as food. That is one of the reasons why our adult vitamin supplements do not say "Keep out of the reach of children."

Let's consider some of the proven benefits of taking these high quality vitamins.

Surveys show that people live longer and have fewer sick days when they take quality vitamins. I would call that a fantastic benefit. One study showed a 25 percent reduced need for cataract surgery for people who take multivitamins, and there are many other similar health benefits. One study showed that people who took good vitamins had only eighteen sick days a year in contrast to an average of thirty-two sick days for non-vitamin takers.

I have heard antagonists say to someone who has a cold, "You have a cold and you take vitamins." Colds do not last as long for those who take good vitamins, but if we don't take the correct type of vitamins, it will take longer for the body to kill that virus or bacteria. If you are taking the right kind of nutrients, you can speed up the response of your immune system so the cold doesn't last as long. This is true for allergies and sinuses or any other immune response.

Let's consider some other reasons why we need good supplementation based on science and research:

What about cancer prevention? Cancer is the most dreaded health issue. Everybody dreads hearing those words: "We have bad news for you. You have cancer." **A study was done on the antioxidant trace mineral selenium. It almost wiped out every form of cancer and showed a dramatic reduction in most forms of cancer.**

We need organic selenium; however, most sources of selenium are inorganic. The organic source is the only one that provides the health benefit. Many times, vitamin companies showcase the name selenium on their labels, but they are not giving us the type of nutrient that provides the best health benefits. And why are we taking these in the first place if it isn't to get healthier?

We have a million or more Americans who are deficient in B12. There was a recent study that showed elderly women would avoid hearing loss if they would just get more vitamin B12 in their diets. Examine your vitamin bottles, and most say six micrograms. It needs to be three hundred micrograms or more and needs to be absorbable. You also need to take it along with a high potency vitamin B complex. You never single out a B vitamin. God gave us the complete B complex, which is composed of eight vitamins in the right combination. If you single out a B vitamin, it will begin to pull from other areas of the body to find balance.

Why do most manufacturers not make the perfect multi? Because it costs too much money to do it right. Consumers are cost sensitive. However, we spend more money on dog food, cat food, hamburgers, candy, and potato chips than on quality vitamins. To get some good coverage, you will probably have to spend at least a dollar a day to begin to get in the nutrients you need.

Some multivitamin bottles are $68; others run to $98. The multi that we recommend costs anywhere from $18 to $30 depending on the age group. We carry the most complete multivitamins in the world, and they work . . . they actually break down in the bloodstream and don't stop up the plumbing as so many do. *We offer a multivita-min-mineral for all ages from the cradle to the grave!* Twenty-four percent of Americans are taking vitamins on a regular basis; about 70 percent now and then. Of the 24 percent who take the vitamins, many are taking Centrum, Theragram M, or Flintstone vitamins, which are incomplete synthetic vitamins. They are neither potent enough nor really a health product at all. They are synthetic and made with coal tar derivatives. Many fall prey to advertisements by business people who advertise on television "the most complete vitamin for men or for women." These are not health companies at all.

Below are common questions we hear a lot from people. Supple-mentation is such an important subject, and I know it can be confus-ing to figure out what you should be taking and why. There's a lot of marketing hype out there, and it's hard to hear the truth through all that clutter.

Question:
I eat pretty well most of the time and try to eat fruits and vegeta-bles. Why do I even need supplements?
Answer:
That's great that you try to eat healthy most of the time, and that is what I advise everyone to do. However, sadly, it is almost impossible to get all the nutrients you need day in and day out just from the food you eat. If you eat fast food, if you are dieting, or if you skip meals from time to time (and we all do that now and then), it makes it even harder. Plus, it's true that 80 percent of us don't eat the recommended

seven to nine servings of fruits and vegetables that we need each day. And so many snacks which are marketed as healthy options are filled with sugar, fat, and artificial ingredients. Even the fruits and vegetables that we do eat may not be as rich in nutrients as we think. In fact, a recent study of forty-three crops showed a decline in the nutrient content over the past fifty years. So try as we might, the fact is that the vast majority of us don't get all the nutrients we need from the food we eat. So, at the very least, I believe we should all consider taking a foundational multivitamin supplement. This is essential for any health plan.

Studies that have found that long-term supplement users have a 73 percent lower risk of having diabetes as compared to the individuals who use no supplements. The multiple supplement group also had a 39 percent lower risk of high blood pressure as compared to the no supplement group. And those who took multiple supplements long term had a 33 percent lower triglyceride level on average as compared to the group who didn't take supplements.

Why is this important? Because high triglyceride levels have been linked to atherosclerosis, and by extension, the risk for heart disease and stroke. This group also had a 59 percent lower level of C-reactive protein, which is the measure of inflammation in comparing to the group that did not supplement. We know that those with elevated levels of C-reactive protein are at increased risk of many diseases including diabetes, high blood pressure, and cardiovascular disease.

Question:

Aren't all vitamins the same? Why should I spend more for one brand when there are low-cost vitamins at places like Costco?

Answer:

This is a great question. Remember that old adage "You get what you pay for"? I think it definitely applies here. First of all, I suggest you look for a reputable company that bases its formulations on sound science and efficacy, as most do not. However, this is essential for your health. Again, there is a lot of hype out there.

Secondly, you should look for a company that also has policies in place for monitoring the purity and the potency of its ingredients. High quality ingredients and strict testing policies cost money. So these pure and effective products will tend to cost more. Too often, discounted brands will use lower quality ingredients and fillers to keep the price low. Another problem with some discount brands is that their supplements are not always sufficiently absorbed by the body. So even though the label may say the supplement contains, for example, 100 percent of the nutrient, it may not be dissolving properly, so your body may not actually be absorbing that amount of that nutrient. One more warning about cheaper brands: you are not always getting the full spectrum of vitamins and minerals at optimum levels. Take, for example, the B vitamins, where the percentage of daily value is sometimes absurdly low. Another example is the supplement that only provides you with one kind of vitamin E as opposed to the full spectrum of tocopherols that we know are associated with good health.

Question:

Heart disease runs in my family. I am always struggling to manage my cholesterol. Can supplements help?

Answer:

They certainly can. Supplements containing plant sterols and stanols have been shown to reduce cholesterol levels. In fact, there is enough evidence for the benefit of these ingredients that even the FDA is on board by allowing a heart health claim for products that meet specific requirements with plant sterols and stanols. Individuals who take multiple supplements over a long period of time have an 11 percent lower ratio of total cholesterol in addition to the lower level of triglycerides and C-reactive protein that I mentioned earlier.

I also want to mention the heart health benefits of what I think is one of the most important supplements that we all should be taking every day. This is omega-3 fatty acids. According to the American Heart Association, omega-3 fatty acids help decrease triglyceride levels, slow the growth rate of atherosclerotic plaque, and lower blood pressure. I recommend quality fish oil capsules encapsuled for freshness. This is another product that we offer.

Question:

Everyone in my office seems to be coming down with colds and the flu; I can't afford to be sick again. I'm almost out of sick days. I've heard vitamin C helps. Is that true?

Answer:

The cold and flu season can be especially bad some years. People get colds and the flu because they are sick internally. So it is very important to keep your immune system healthy. Stress and lack of rest can be factors as well. Keeping your immune system healthy is very important. Supplementing daily with antioxidants like vitamin E, vitamin C, beta carotene and other carotenoids, zinc, and selenium are very important for bolstering your immune system. Also, make sure you are getting plenty of vitamin D3 every day. And when you are feeling especially at risk, make sure you increase the amount of vitamin C, zinc, and selenium you are taking and add some echinacea to the mix. Again, any information I am suggesting with regard to supplementation is based on the supplements we carry. We know the science and efficacy pertaining to those supplements.

Question:

It just seems like I'm tired all the time. I have no energy and no spark. Work and kids are wearing me out. Can supplements help me get my energy back?

Answer:

Yes, taking daily supplements is a great start toward becoming a more energized you. It's amazing what happens when you give your body what it needs to run efficiently. The B vitamins, especially B12, are extremely important for both energy and mood. According to the National Institutes of Health, up to 15 percent of us may have a vitamin B12 deficiency, which can lead to fatigue, weakness, memory issues, hearing issues, and mood swings. Along with vitamin B12, you always need to take the complete B complex. There are also studies that suggest that the omega-3 fatty acids can also have a very positive impact on both energy and mood as well. So take your vitamins, and also get plenty of exercise and try to get more sleep. That plan will help reduce your stress and pick up your energy level.

Question:

My problem is with my skin. It doesn't have that healthy glow any more. I've tried topical creams that have not worked. I am wondering if it has more to do with the nutrition I am getting or not getting.

Answer:

I think sometimes we forget that the healthy glow we all want to have really has to come from the inside out. And there are specific nutrients that contribute to healthy skin. Vitamin C is critical for collagen formation, which helps with the firmness of the skin. And vitamin E helps protect the lipids in our skin. One of the best things you can do to help keep that healthy glow is to avoid oxidative damage from things like sun exposure, poor diet (especially fatty foods), excess alcohol consumption, smoking, and being exposed to environmental pollution. But damage from the sun is really the number one cause of skin aging, so wear your sunscreen. Also consider supplementing with carotenoids such as beta carotene and lycopene, which actually have been shown to give a little bit of extra UV protection to your skin. You will see creams advertise that they contain some of these vitamins as ingredients because they actually can have a positive impact on your skin. But just remember, it's much more important to get these nutrients daily so they can work from the inside out.

Question:

I used to be able to eat anything, but not anymore. I just wonder if there is some sort of vitamin that can help me get my digestion back in shape.

Answer:

As we all know, healthy digestion is essential to insure that your body can absorb all the nutrients you need as well as pass the toxins through. So it is important to pay attention when things get a little bit out of whack. But it doesn't take much, unfortunately. Changes in our diet, stress, and lots of other things can throw the micro flora in your digestive system out of balance. I recommend that everyone take both the pre- and the probiotic daily to help maintain healthy bacteria in your intestines.

Question:
Will supplements help me live longer?
Answer:
Just think of the top killers in our nation. Long-term supplement users have lower risk factors for all the top diseases out there. Your body contains trillions of cells, and billions of new cells are created every day. Each and every cell is like a high performance engine. It needs high quality raw materials (nutrients) to function properly. And these nutrients affect every system of our body. Truly, how you look, feel, and perform is directly affected by your nutrient intake. So for living longer, studies show that if you've got the nutrients you need, maintain a healthy weight, and exercise regularly, you greatly reduce your risk of developing serious diseases. And one of the ways to make sure you are getting what you need consistently is through proper supplementation.

Question:
I'd rather be focusing on eating healthy foods than taking a bunch of pills. I think that is the most natural way to get the nutrients I need. And wouldn't it be less expensive in the long run than taking a lot of supplements?
Answer:
I couldn't agree more. We should be eating more fresh fruits and vegetables and more lean protein sources like chicken and fish and avoiding unhealthy fats, fast foods, and packaged foods that contain lots of sugar and preservatives. But with our hectic lifestyles, it's just not that easy to do. In fact a study of over four thousand Americans showed that at least 50 percent of the individuals surveyed who obtain the nutrients from food alone fell below the estimated average

requirements for vitamins A, B, and E. For those individuals who use supplements along with food to obtain their nutrients, less than 10 percent fell below those requirements. If you want to talk about value, let's talk about how much food you would have to buy and eat to get the recommended amounts of just a couple of nutrients. For example, vitamin D3 is a nutrient that we now know impacts so many areas of our health. To get the recommended amount of vitamin D, you would have to drink five cups of cow's milk per day. Who's going to do that? As for B complex, you'd have to eat six cups of spinach a day to meet your folate or B complex needs. And what about omega-3s from fish? We would have to eat four servings of omega-3-rich fish a week to meet the one gram a day amount. The point is that in our busy lives, it can be very difficult to eat the way we should.

So eat the Bible-nutritional way (this was and still is God's perfect diet), and take your very selective supplements every day.

I want to emphasize, too, how important it is to buy your supplements from a reputable company. To make sure you are getting the best quality ingredients available, look for a company that focuses on safety and quality and one that publishes clinical studies on its ingredients and products, especially in peer-review journals. As for the ingredients, you want supplements with natural ingredients whenever possible without artificial flavors, sweeteners, or preservatives added. We can offer the best. Call us if you need help with this at (972) 380-5363.

In conclusion, chemical vitamins do unhealthy things to your body. In contrast, unaltered food supplements do healthy things for the body. Isn't your body worth the best?

When buying a brand of supplements:

- Look for clinical studies on the ingredients in that respective bottle.
- Look for natural ingredients on the label like food: alfalfa, fish oil, etc.
- Avoid artificial sweeteners, flavors, and preservatives.
- Look for a company that focuses on safety, efficacy, and quality and has the clinical research to prove it.

Have you been given a diagnosis? If so, it doesn't have to be fatal.

I personally know how scary it can be when your body is out of control. I do not believe that the diagnosis you have been given has to be fatal. There have been many people who have been close to death who have applied these principles of thinking positively, exercising when possible, and applying the proven therapies as given here nutritionally have experienced the miraculous in quality of health and a long healthy life. I believe you can do it, too.

If you have any concerns about your health or want to get on a program for prevention, I encourage you to give our office a call. You can set a phone consultation if you are not in Dallas. The phone number is (972) 380-5363. If you are in the Dallas/Fort Worth area, you can call and set up a time to come into the office and talk about your concerns. We have worked with thousands who now have a quality of health they never thought possible. I am able to counsel you on the foods that will heal your body of whatever concerns you. I will also counsel you on the foods that are contributing to your problem or problems. And because we cannot get what we need in our foods alone today, I will write out the supplements that you need to take, how to take each one, when to take it, and so on. And this is all done for your specific diagnosis or condition. We take the guesswork out of it for you. When you walk out of our office or when you get off the phone, you will know exactly how to take charge of your condition based on my years of working successfully with others. If you are purchasing your supplements from a health food store, you do not have a true professional helping you with your health.

For generalities, I like to recommend what I call the *Better Health Package,* from which everyone can benefit.

I encourage everyone to kick-start their day with a *delicious protein smoothie.* This gets your brain functioning optimally. This is not just any protein powder. Ours are non-GMO and processed with water (not alcohol) and with low heat. That means that the enzymes and the life in that product are still intact. We need vegetable protein, which is much more bioavailable for the body than animal protein. The Cattlemen's Association will not be advertising that. It takes meat seventy-two hours to break down, and many times, it putrefies in the intestines. This can cause many digestive issues.

We need protein to repair, restore, and re-energize on the cellular level and build the immune system. We need this kind of protein to get our brains functioning first thing in the morning. Our protein powders come in vanilla, chocolate, strawberry, peach, or coffee flavor. Use this protein to make a delicious smoothie every morning to kick-start your day and your brain! I love the coffee-flavored one blended with chocolate almond milk and ice. Our brains need complete protein, not just another bowl of shredded wheat or Cheerios drenched in cow's milk. Processed cereals turn to sugar and are stored as fat. Despite what you see advertised on television, Cheerios and other cereals are not clinically tested to normalize cholesterol levels.

A multi–mineral vitamin tablet, like the one we carry, is the most complete one on the market and has stood the test of time for over fifty years. We have this multi for babies, toddlers, children, teenagers, all adults, and for people over fifty years old . . . *from the cradle to the grave.*

The delicious protein powder and the multivitamins are the perfect combination for a *Better Health Starter Package.* You can get them at wholesale pricing, and we drop ship all over the US. You can also order for yourself once we put you in the system. That way, you are operating under the umbrella of *Take Charge of Your Health: A Biblical Perspective.*

Let us know if you would like to order from us. There is a one-time fee of $19.95 to get the wholesale prices. If you want to just start taking what we carry that you are already on, we can do that if you tell us what you are already taking.

If you are not sure of what you need, you will need to set a consultation. We take the guesswork out of it for you. A consultation enables me to give you informed counsel based on knowledge. Are you worth it?

I'd love to be able to help you,

Lilli

Please call (972) 380-5363

Nutritional Deficiency Questionnaire:

B complex Deficiency:
- Fatigue, anemia, insomnia, hair loss, acne, poor digestion, constipation, nervousness

Vitamin C Deficiency:
- Infections, bleeding gums, black and blue marks, hardening of the arteries, nosebleeds

Calcium Deficiency:
- Irritability, muscle cramps, headaches, insomnia, calcium is a natural tranquilizer, bone formation, arthritis, bad teeth, bursitis, backaches, menstrual cramps, soft nails

Vitamin E Deficiency:
- Poor circulation, phlebitis, varicose veins, gangrene, hot flashes, muscular and menstrual cramps, diabetes, heart attack, thrombosis, blood clots, cholesterol buildup, lack of oxygen, premature aging, migraines

Lecithin Deficiency:
- High blood pressure, thrombosis, heart attack, bad memory, poor concentration, kidney disorders, liver issues, bad skin, obesity, nervousness, cholesterol buildup

Magnesium Deficiency:
- Magnesium is involved in three hundred reactions in the body that promote health. Deficiency symptoms are muscle cramps, fatigue, weakness, twitching, and more

Zinc Deficiency:
- Inactive pancreas (from diabetes and alcohol), dry skin, frequent colds, virus infection, no appetite, no taste for foods, chronic infections (take no more than 80 mg daily)

Vitamin D3 Deficiency:

•Weak bones, fractures, prone to colds and flu, rickets, fatigue, depression, joint and muscle pain, chronic pain in body, restless sleep, etc.

CHAPTER 9

The Benefits of Choosing Life

I have heard often that we have no control over when we die because God has numbered our days. If that is so, why would **HE** say we have a choice?

God certainly knows the beginning from the end and knows how long we will live, but He has given us a choice. The message of this book is all about better choices for living long and well on the earth.

Deuteronomy 30:19 (English Standard Version): "I call heaven and earth to witness against you today, that I have set before you life and death, blessing and curse. Therefore, choose life that you and your offspring may live." We can choose, and by now, you should know how to choose and how to make better choices when you go to the grocery store or when you order vitamin supplements.

We need to make wise investments. If we are spending money on supplements, we can now choose to spend our money on ones we know are clinically tested to work for us. Whomever you are giving your money to for supplements should also be qualified to help you with food choices that can save your life and with your health in general.

Studies show that just the simple addition of a quality pure food multivitamin supplement has the following benefits:

- 50 percent reduction of strokes
- 57 percent reduction of high blood pressure
- 21 percent reduction of myocardial infarction (heart attack) in men and 34 percent in women
- 32 percent reduced risk of arterial disease (based on a study of forty-six thousand health professionals)
- 70 percent reduced risk of one of our top killers, colon cancer (the more years of past supplementation, the greater reduction of risk)
- 45 percent reduction of colorectal cancer
- 31 percent reduction of all disease (based on a new study of thirteen thousand men and women with C, E, selenium, and zinc)
- 37 percent reduction of all forms of mortality risk (based on a new study)
- 50 percent reduction of days of infectious disease (based on a study of immune system, improved T killer cells, lymphocytes, interleukin 2, antibodies, all significantly improved with organic multi-vitamins, not synthetic)
- 82 percent reduction of incidence of infection in type 2 diabetes and 100 percent reduction of missed work if taking organic multivitamins
- 42 percent reduction risk of MS (based on a brand new vitamin D3 study)
- 28 percent reduction of rheumatoid arthritis in women and 34–35 percent in men
- 70 percent decline in neural tube birth defects
- 30 percent reduction in neuroblastoma (nerve cell tumors in children) if multi taken in early pregnancy; 40 percent reduction if supplement in second and third trimesters
- 85 percent reduction in diabetic-associated birth defects in women with diabetes (Source: Jean Mayer, USDA Human Research

Center on Aging; and Jeffrey Blumberg, PhD, FACN, CNS; professor of the Friedman School of Nutrition Science and Policy; associate director and chief, Antioxidants Research Lab, Tufts University.)

When you give the body what it needs, it can do all of the above **and more.**

Here's the "More"

- Your body is able to reproduce a new liver in just six months.
- Your cells are able to reproduce and become totally new in just eleven months.
- Every ounce of bone in your body can become totally new in just two years.
- Every blood cell can rejuvenate and become new in just eleven months.

What can we do to protect and improve our health? It's not always difficult if you know what to observe. Begin to read labels carefully, and don't eat foods with a lot of added salt. Eat more fresh fruits and vegetables. That will give you a lot of potassium. Try to keep your sodium intake to less than one thousand milligrams a day (most Americans consume between eight thousand to ten thousand milligrams of sodium a day; our ancestors ate about seven hundred milligrams a day). Excess salt can cause a lot of damage to your health. Many do not realize that eating too much salt can cause the body to lose calcium, which contributes to osteoporosis. You will naturally eat more potassium if you eat more fresh fruits and vegetables. But beware even in a health food store. Look at the label on one slice of so-called healthy bread. It can contain as much as three hundred milligrams of sodium. That means three thin slices could give you the maximum sodium for the day. As much as possible, eat plant-based foods that are organic and fresh. Try to eat them raw. You can choose to eat a salad instead of a cheeseburger. You can choose to drink mineral water instead of a soft drink. Remember, soft drinks produce soft bones. You can choose fruit for a snack instead of a candy bar. You can substitute a vegetable for French fries. You can choose brown rice instead of white rice. And the fruit of all these good choices will have a very positive impact on your health, just as the cumulative effect of all our bad choices has a negative effect. What can we do about this?

You don't have to eat bad food. What you eat is within your control to choose.

The human body, being created by God, is the healer. It is an amazing machine when we treat it right.

With all of this science, the case for supplementation with at least an organic multivitamin is convincing. Everyone should take a multi every day consistently, **not just hit or miss.** If you are spending money on vitamins, you might as well take them in a consistent way.

CHAPTER 10

Living Long and Well on the Earth

If God Says Our Days Are Numbered, Do We Have Any Choice in the Matter?

Do you ever hear conversations like this? *Is this your experience?*

"I've sure gotten old! I've had two bypass surgeries, a hip replacement, new knees, I'm half blind, can't hear anything quieter than a jet engine, I take forty different medications that make me dizzy, winded, and subject to blackouts. I have bouts of dementia. I have poor circulation; I can hardly feel my hands and feet anymore. I can't remember if I am eighty-five or ninety-five. I've lost all my friends. But, thank God, I still have my driver's license!"

Or this?

"I can live with my arthritis, my bifocals fit me fine, my teeth are quite comfortable but, oh, how I miss my mind!"

Do you ever hear conversations like that? It can be all too often, sadly.

The following are some examples in the Bible, however, of people who lived godly and long lives.

What about Moses?
Did he die sick?
The Scripture says that he died at 120, and his eyes were not dim and his vigor was not abated (Deuteronomy 34:7).

What about Joshua?
Did he die sick?
The Scripture says he was still active and died at 110 . . . (Joshua 24:29).

What about Caleb?
Caleb was well able to take the mountain at age eighty-five . . . (Joshua 14:12).

He said, "Give me this mountain. The Lord has kept me alive these forty-five years since the Lord spoke to Moses. *I am today eighty-five years old; yet, I am as strong* today as I was then" (Joshua 14:10-12). Caleb had received the promise. He walked in wholeness and godliness and humility. He asked for the mountain but knew it would take God to conquer and He did.

How long do you want to live? How long do you want to live in health? How long can you live? I have heard pastors say, "We have no control over how long we will live or when we will die."

Read the following Scriptures and see how that statement does **not** line up with God's heart and His truth about life and death. Just because God's Word says "Our days are numbered" does not mean that while we are here we don't have some control over how long those days will be. God has given us a free will and power to choose life or death. If we line up with His will, we will be ordering our lifestyle choices to prolong our days and not shorten them. This is called wisdom. Health is a choice.

I had a well-meaning woman come up to me after a seminar and say, "Lilli, how am I supposed to die if I never get sick?" What she did not realize is that sickness is the way of the world. God's plan for His children is that we not get sick. We don't have to get sick to die. When we are fully satisfied, God just takes us home in our sleep. This is what is happening in many other cultures that are eating the foods God told us to eat. That was Moses and Joshua's experience.

What does God's Word say? Does God promise health and long life? We must be fully convinced in our hearts and mind that it is God's will for us to be well. If you are not convinced, your mind will yield to sickness and to satanic forces, and you will not walk in His health. And many then yield to the three score and ten mindset, which is the lifespan of the world and Egypt, and consequently, the diseases of the world and Egypt.

Let us consider these promises and allow them to take deep root in our hearts and move out of the realm of opinion to a deep-hearted conviction.

It is written:	Proverbs 3:1, 2 – "My son do not forget my law; but let your heart keep my commandments; *for length of days, long life, and peace* shall they add to you." (emphasis mine)
It is written:	Proverbs 4:10 – "Hear, my son, attend to my words, and *your years of life will be many.*" (emphasis mine)
It is written:	Psalms 105:37 – "He brought them out with silver and gold and not one among them was feeble."
It is written:	Deuteronomy 5:33 – "You shall walk in the ways of the Lord that you may live and that it may be well with you and that you may *prolong your days in the land* which you shall possess." (emphasis mine)
It is written:	Psalms 91:16 – "*With long life* [emphasis mine] I will satisfy him and show him my salvation." (NIV)

It is written: Psalms 92:14-16 – "Growing in grace *they shall still bring forth fruit in their OLD AGE*; they shall be full of sap and vitality. They will be living memorials. With long life I will show him my salvation." (Amplified; emphasis mine)

It is written: Psalms 92:4 – "Let us go on and grow in grace and bring forth very positive fruit *in our old age and be living memorials* of God's goodness and how He is faithful to His promises." (emphasis mine)

It is written: Proverbs 4:22 – "My word is life and health to a man's whole body."

It is written: Deuteronomy 7:14-15 – "You will be a blessed people. None of your men or women will be childless and the Lord will keep you free from *every disease*." (emphasis mine)

It is written: Deuteronomy 33:25 – "The bolts of your gates will be iron and bronze *and your strength will be equal to your days*." (emphasis mine)

It is written: Joshua 14:11 – *"I am as strong today as I was the day Moses sent me*: as my strength was then, *so is my strength now*, for war and to go out and come in." (emphasis mine)

It is written: Ruth 4:15 – *"He will renew your life and sustain you in your old age."* (emphasis mine)

It is written: Job 5:26 – *"You will come to the grave in old age."* (emphasis mine)

It is written: Psalms 103:5 – "He satisfies my mouth with good things [food] so that my *youth is renewed like the eagles*." (emphasis mine)

It is written: Genesis 6:3 – *"Man's days will be 120 years."* (emphasis mine)

It is written: Psalms 90:10 – The days of our years are three score and ten." The footnote here says, "This was considered to be a curse, God intended man *to live to be 120."* (emphasis mine)

I wish you the very best of health for at least one hundred years and beyond, and the only way that can happen is to build your immune system with proper nutrients and saturate your mind with the truth.

If you feel the need for a one-on-one consultation about your health concerns or just want to know what to do to prevent disease and know how to avoid the slippery slope, please give me a call and set a consultation time on the calendar at (972) 380-5363.

After you do a consultation with us, we give a monthly free follow-up if you are using our supplements. This is a real blessing. We want to give you the support you need. Most feel the need for this. We approach health issues from a biblical perspective and the latest of cutting edge in science and so our ministry is really a win-win for you.

I wish you the best of health and a long and very satisfying life. I hope this book has been an eye-opener and an inspiration to you. Please forward this information on to others across the nation. It has literally saved thousands of lives, including my own. You just don't hear this information enough. Remember, it is difficult to accomplish much or enjoy much in life if you don't feel well.

David said, "With God's help, I can run against a troop and leap over a wall" (Psalm18:29). This is a physical declaration, not just a spiritual one. We will need strong knees, hips, and joints to do this. God is calling us to battle and to climb mountains!

We will need these physical weapons in addition to our spiritual weapons for warfare, climbing mountains, and running against troops.

Come on, let's go and get into the battle fully equipped: body, soul, and spirit! We were born and called for *VICTORY*!

Paul says in I Corinthians 6:19-20, "What? Know ye not that your body is the temple of the Holy Ghost which is in you, which ye have of God and you are not your own? You have been bought with a price: therefore, glorify God in your body, and in your spirit, which are God's."

Another Important Vitamin

Have you ever heard about vitamin L?

When it comes to vitamins, I want to acquaint you with a very important one.

I love to call it "vitamin L." I want you to take a dose of vitamin L every day. Don't miss even one dose. Just as with vitamin D and its newest research, we need a lot more of vitamin L. You will be amazed at what it can do for you. To confirm my point, the Scripture teaches that laughter is like a medicine. It's a good medicine without toxic side effects . . . only benefits. Your doctor may not have prescribed this. You know, it's free. The joy of the Lord is your strength. And so I call this vitamin L for laughter.

The latest research says that laughter is a wonderful medicine because it causes the release of body chemicals called endorphins. These substances help to relieve pain and create a sense of well-being. Laughter increases blood flow as much as exercise does. Laughter raises your energy level and pulls you out of the pit of depression. Laughter releases tension, anxiety, anger, fear, shame, and guilt and can completely change a person's attitude. Laughter strengthens your immune system. It increases antibodies. It is believed to have a protective capacity against viruses, bacteria, and other microorganisms. It's an internal aerobic exercise. You inhale more oxygen when you laugh. Laughter stimulates your heart and blood circulation as an equivalent to any other standard aerobic exercise.

The first documented case of humor positively affecting disease was in 1964 when Norman Cousins published *Anatomy of an Illness*. Medical professionals for the first time were shown that humor biologically reversed Cousins' ankylosing spondylitis, a painful disease causing the disintegration of the spinal connective tissue. Given a one in five hundred chance of recovery, Cousins decided to infuse himself with *humor treatments*. His wife would buy funny videos for him to enjoy.

With Cousin's self-designed *humor treatments,* he found that fifteen minutes of hearty laughter could produce two hours of pain free sleep. Blood samples also showed that his inflammation level was lowered after the humor treatments. Eventually, Cousins was able to completely reverse the illness. Cousins later documented his story in his book.

Dr. Lee Berk and fellow researcher Dr. Stanley Tan of Loma Linda University in California have been studying the effects of laughter on the immune system. To date their published studies have shown that laughing lowers blood pressure, reduces stress hormones, increases muscle flexion, and boosts immune function by raising levels of infection-fighting T cells, disease-fighting proteins called gamma interferon and B-cells, which produce disease destroying antibodies. Laughter also triggers the release of endorphins and produces a general sense of well-being. This is very good for the human body. There is a summary of his research published in the September/October 1996 issue of the *Humor and Health Journal.*

So as you begin a new journey, don't forget to lighten up and laugh. Don't be so serious about everything. The Scripture says "take no thought" about worry and anxiety, and that really helps with stress and high blood pressure. Remember, Jesus was into celebrations, fun, and laughter, and we need to be, too. When you laugh, it simply makes you feel good, and that is very healthy. I really like that!

Inspirational Authors on this Topic

Dr. Ted Broer
Maximum Energy

Elmer A. Josephson
God's Key to Health and Happiness

T. Colin Campbell, PhD
The China Study

Gary Null, PhD with Martin Feldman, MD; Deborah Raslo, MD, and Carolyn Dean, MD, ND
Death by Medicine

Raymond Francis, MSc
Never Be Sick Again

Dr. Gordon S. Tessler
The Genesis Diet

Disclaimer:

Please note: The information in this book is for educational purposes only. It should not be used as a substitute for appropriate medical advice, nor should any information in it be interpreted as prescriptive. This information is based on years of study and research and is the result of helping thousands achieve optimal health over the last thirty years.

About Lilli Taylor Hetherington

Lilli is a global spokeswoman for walking in health. Few have experienced her success in working with people across the nation with cancer, heart disease, diabetes, osteoporosis, arthritis and all degenerative diseases. These are the diseases that are coming from what we put in our bodies. She knows what the body needs to prevent, heal, and walk in health for many years. She knows what the body needs to have more energy. It is no mystery to her what the cause and cure of cancer is, for example. Her work and message has touched thousands across the globe and has stood the test of time now for nearly forty years.

She has long been affiliated with 100.7 FM KWRD in Dallas, Texas. Hundreds of her patient/clients share their health testimonies daily on KWRD.

This book is about prevention. *Early detection* is one thing, but *prevention* is better.

Lilli has devoted her professional life to educating Americans in how to take charge of their own health and their future. All of her nutritional programs are from the latest of cutting-edge science as well as from a biblical perspective. Few nutrition books have this unique combination and success.

The current model in our nation on health is not sustainable. ***This book covers the key areas of prevention.***

Lilli is a former Hollywood model; she is a professional singer, speaker, and author. Most of all, she is a godly wife, mother, and now grandmother.

At the University of Texas, she met the man of her dreams and the man of God's choice for her. Together they were directors with Campus Crusade for Christ (now called Cru), for several years until God led James into commercial real estate in Dallas. Lilli lives in Dallas, Texas, with her husband. James and Lilli have two wonderful sons and ten grandchildren. Lilli's greatest credentials are the hundreds or possibly thousands of people who have been influenced positively by her work and care.

If you have been given a diagnosis, Lilli has a large nutritional counseling practice and can help you back to health. If you just want to prevent, she can help you with her program for prevention. Although she is located in Dallas, Texas, she works with people regularly all across the nation. If they are too far to come into the office, they can do phone consultations, and the cost is all the same. *Call (972) 380-5363 to set an appointment.*

It is pretty difficult to find this unique package just anywhere. Lilli saves her clients many dollars. Many have been just "out there," navigating the Internet by themselves and simply hoping and guessing. This lacks the personal touch. When you do a consultation with Lilli, she will provide you a list of foods that can prevent or heal your body of that condition. She will also list the foods that contribute to that problem, just so you know. Because you can't get what you need in your foods alone today, she will list the selective organic supplements you need for that condition, how to take them, what each one is for, and when to take it. When you walk out of her office, you will know exactly what to do to take charge of that condition based on her many years of helping people. She takes the "guesswork" out of it for you. If you are buying from a health food store, you simply cannot get the kind of wise counsel that comes from years of successfully working with people. Her help and counsel is truly a win-win for you! *Call (972) 380-5363.*

Your Prayer of Surrender (Romans 12)

Father, in the name of Jesus, I recommit my life to you: body, soul, and spirit. I cannot do this without You. As my mind has now been renewed with Your truth and my eyes have been opened, I ask you to give me the motivation I need to apply Your truth. I ask You to grant me an overwhelming desire to walk in Your wonderful ways of health, vitality, and the abundant life in order to fulfill Your callings on my life for many years to come.

In Jesus's name and for the Kingdom's sake,
Amen

I want to congratulate you on finding this cutting-edge information that you need to get healthy and stay healthy. All of this information is from the latest of cutting-edge science as well as from a Biblical perspective. In other words, it is a win-win for you.

No one knows better than God how your body and mind is to function optimally.

As the T-shirt says, "**when all else fails, read the manual.**" All else is failing in the area of health, so it is time for us to try out what the manual says. Our Designer and Creator created us with a manual. Unfortunately, we have not been taught what the manual has to say about health and nutrition.

I am so excited that you are reading this book. I truly believe that a healthy diet and lifestyle (what we eat and what we think) is a cornerstone of overall optimal health.

I work with people daily across the nation in coaching them to a quality of health they never thought possible. Some have been even fourth stage cancer patients, and they are doing well and giving their health testimonies on the radio.

It is amazing how God has created our bodies. They will heal themselves when we give them what they need.

If you are not sure of what you need, please give me a call to set an appointment to visit about a plan of prevention tailor-made for you or a plan for your healing.

I wish you the very best of health,

Lilli Hetherington
I look forward to hearing from you.
www.takechargeofyourhealth.org
(972) 380-5363

Parting Thoughts

I can give you this guarantee:

Good nutrition equals good health.

Poor nutrition equals poor health.

That's pure science.

God's Heart is to bless.

Let's stay under His umbrella of protection and blessing.

It's a choice and a blessing.

You don't want to miss out on this.

Don't wait for a diagnosis.

The choices we make in our daily food selections can totally prevent our top killers.

I trust your choice will be blessings and wonderful health for the long haul!

Printed in the USA
CPSIA information can be obtained
at www.ICGtesting.com
JSHW012031140824
68134JS00033B/2990